The complete food makeover

This book is dedicated to my mum, Kay, the fabbest of them all.
She taught me all the best things I know.
Everyday, her light and love inspires me and all those around her.
And for that, I am truly greatful.

Thank you to the many people who helped and supported me through the *Complete Food Makeover* journey. Mum for the many hours of recipe testing she gave me, Dad for his never ending willingness to taste the desserts, Judy for her sharp editing eye, Peter for his humour, Lisa Reid for her excellent troubleshooting skills and support, Lisa Rishmiller for calling at just the right time, Jo Mackay for her belief in me and her commitment to a quality product and Justin and the boys for allowing me to write, create and be me.

A final thank you to all of you, who bought this book, and are brave enough to make changes to the way you eat and live. The rewards will be enormous.

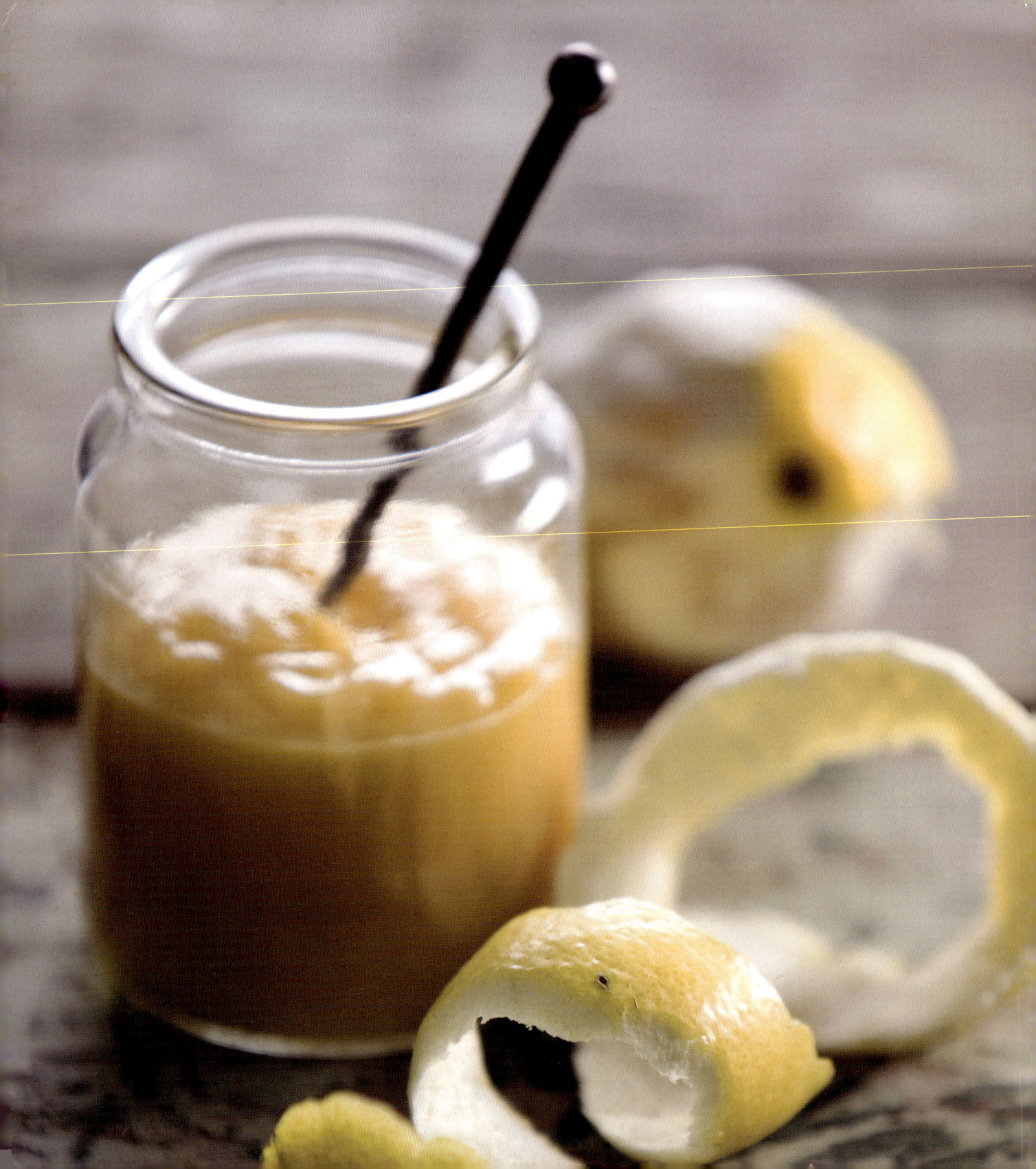

The complete food makeover

Julie Maree Wood

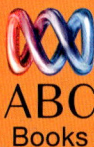

ABC
Books

Contents

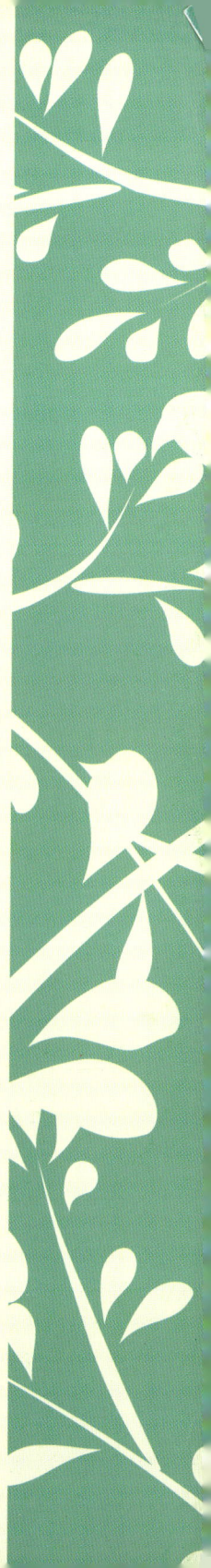

Introduction

This is not a diet book, it's a makeover book for food. It's filled with recipes that taste like the old comfort food favourites (some of them taste even better) but they have been nipped, tucked and boosted to get them working harder for you.

It's for people who want to eat well but just can't resist fast, fatty food. Naughty but nice we like to call it and we all love it. There's nothing like hot chips and sauce, a couple of 'bite-sized' sausage rolls, some crunchy, cheesy nachos on your lap in front of the TV or a few slices of pizza on a Friday night. It's not just a comforting treat, it's fun and it's delicious.

Let's take the guilt out of these lovely pleasures by making a few simple changes, giving your fat faves a makeover and transforming them from fat to fab. They'll still taste delicious but will no longer have all of those hidden nasties, so there will be no need to feel guilty after indulging in them. A boost of iron here, a shot of fibre there, a trim of fat or a cut in sugar. Whether you make all of the fab changes or only one or two, it all makes a difference. Your body will love it and your tastebuds will never know the difference.

Of course these delicious fat-to-fab menu favourites are not the cornerstone of a good diet. Relatively healthy as they may be, the fab version of sausage rolls will still add to your waistline if you munch on them for lunch everyday. A fab recipe once or twice a week is enough to tantalise your tastebuds but still keep you looking foxy.

Finally, some food your tastebuds and your heart can agree on.

Julie Maree Wood

How to use this book

This book's list of recipes reads more like a takeaway menu than a healthy eating book, that's because *The Complete Food Makeover*, or as I like to call it, *Fat to Fab* is written for everyone who loves to indulge in traditionally unhealthy food but wants to make a modern healthy version that is kind to your body and also satisfies your cravings. Or *you* may be committed to eating well but your family or partner loves their fatty favourites and you are tired of cooking two meals every night. The fab versions of your family's or partner's favourites will keep everyone happy.

It's great if you're looking to makeover your favourite comfort foods as it could be a gateway to giving your diet a bit of an overhaul. If it's not, then skip over the healthy eating tips and tools and just stick with the recipes. Whichever option you choose, it is a step in the right direction. With that in mind, the book is filled with lots of nutrition information, simple ideas to make healthy eating easier, and support to help you achieve whatever your dietary goals are. You may be looking to boost your energy, to feel more vital, to sleep better, lose some weight, to maintain your weight or just to make an effort to eat healthier food but you cannot bear to give up your indulgences.

You can follow the recipes exactly or make just one or two of the changes suggested. The idea is to improve the nutrition of the dishes and *every* change counts, so if you love pasta carbonara but can't stand wholemeal pasta, then make all of the other changes and stick with your white pasta favourite. Just take note of the fibre you're missing out on and boost it in other areas, for example have a high-fibre fruit smoothie for breakfast.

For more recipes, ideas and inspiration visit www.thecompletefoodmakeover.com.au

Five-star rating

All of the recipes have a five-star rating on the top of the page. This rating is to give you an idea of just how healthy the makeover recipe is and how it can fit into your everyday diet. Ninety percent of the original 'fat' recipes would have received no stars if they were rated but the fab recipes range from three stars to the full five stars. Here's how to use the five-star ratings.

★★★ 3 stars – Good for a treat or on a special occasion.

★★★★ 4 stars – There are lots of healthy things to offer in these recipes.
Serve them with a five-star side to win back that extra star.

★★★★★ 5 stars – This is a five-star makeover.

For a complete meal

At the bottom of many recipes suggestions are given for what to serve with the dish to ensure that you have a complete nutritional meal.

For food nerds like me

For the food nerds like me, many of the recipes have a very nerdy way to boost the 'healthiness' of the recipe even further. This is noted at the bottom of the recipe. All of the tips are simple and will rarely change the final outcome of the recipe in terms of look or taste. Sometimes the suggestion will be to add a little wheat germ to boost the nutrients, or to reduce the sugar further by adding extra fruit or vegetables, or using other superfoods to boost the nutrition of the dish and make it worthy of a bonus star. The food nerd tips are optional.

Sugar and salt

You will see that some of the recipes use added sugar or salt. How could a naturopath and nutritionist possibly add salt or sugar to a recipe, you might ask? It is impossible to completely avoid these two additives as they do so many wonderful things in cooking. The trick is to minimise them and that is what all of the fab recipes do. They have been reduced to the lowest possible amount needed to get the job done. If you compare the levels of sugar and salt in the fab recipes to their fat counterparts or, better still, the shop bought alternatives, the salt and sugar savings are enormous.

Butter and spreads

None of the recipes use butter as it is so high in saturated fat. In the recipes where a spread is used to replace the butter, the ingredient will be listed as good quality spread. This means spreads that are based on seed oils or olive oil and so are filled with the good fats, not the bad. Spend some time having a look at the different brands of spreads available at the supermarket and choose one that is low in saturated fat, has no trans fats and is low in salt. (Trans fats are bad fats that are produced during processing; they are known to be harmful to the body and so are best minimised in your diet.) You still have to be conservative when using these spreads, as they are still high in fat, but they contain better fat than the saturated fat in butter.

Nutrition panels

At the bottom of each recipe there is a nutrition panel showing the kilojoule, calorie, fat, saturated fat, protein, fibre and carbohydrate content of the recipe. These panels are approximates only but they are included to give you a gauge of what you are consuming. If some of you are on a weight-loss program, they can be a handy tool to use. Perhaps the most interesting aspect of these panels is when you compare the amounts to the amounts in the traditional fat recipes. Where possible, the fat content of the traditional recipe has been added. A couple of the fab recipes may look a little high in some areas until you compare them to the traditional recipe and see the massive savings the makeover gives you.

Halving and doubling

Most of the recipes feed four people but you may live in a household of one or two or you may be feeding six each night. If you are cooking for one or two, you don't need to eat the same meal for four nights in a row. Other than being a poor dietary habit, it is also very boring. To make it easier to halve or double recipes to suit your individual and household needs, please refer to the table on page 244 in Resources at the end of this book. Please note that in these recipes 1 tablespoon equals 15ml *not* 20ml.

A final note

Rigid diets are impossible to sustain as they try to suspend us above the real world. Who has time to weigh their food, count their calories or check their guidebook for what they can and cannot eat? To maintain a healthy weight, keep your energy levels bursting or just feel fantastic, you need a way to be able to eat well all the time, not just when you are trying to keep a new year's resolution or maintain a health kick. *The Complete Food Makeover* is not a diet, it's a way to incorporate healthy eating into the everyday foods you already love and crave. Adding some five-star side dishes is an even better way to boost your favourites and add a couple of extra stars to your fab five-star rating for the meal. Use five-star side dishes regularly and even add some of your own to the mix.

Good on you for taking the time to give your diet a bit of razzle dazzle. It will take no time at all to get into the fab way of doing things and you'll be making over your own recipes to produce your own delicious and nutritious delights. This is a fantastic step in the right direction.

What does healthy diet mean in our chaotic lives?

Busy, busy, busy. It must be the most popular word of the twenty-first century. The more machines we invent to help us, the more we expect of ourselves and our time. How can we possibly eat well when our lives are so chaotic? The question, however, should really be, how can we possibly afford *not* to eat well?

We're all busy, but investing some time and effort into a great diet can be the very thing to propel you forward and help you excel in your busy life. The Western world is racing faster than ever and if you try to run your body on poor fuel, like any racing car, you are going to conk out well before the finish line.

A great diet will reward you in numerous ways. In the short term, you'll feel your energy levels soar, your sleep will often improve, your skin will begin to glow, your moods will be more predictable and so will your bowels. Everybody will ask you what on earth have you been doing to look so drop dead gorgeous! You'll quickly realise how shabby you were feeling when you were eating more fat than fab.

In the longer term, a great diet can reduce your chances of developing serious conditions such as bowel cancer, heart disease, high cholesterol, obesity and Type II diabetes.

You don't need a degree in nutrition or ten hours a day in the kitchen to be able to eat well and you don't need to be a boring food nerd either. What you do need is some basic nutrition knowledge, some commitment to where you want to go, a positive attitude and to know how to spin your favourite fat dishes into a great choice. It's all about balance.

If it sounds like too much, then why not challenge yourself for just two weeks? Work hard to eat really fab food and assess how you feel after the fortnight. If you feel better, commit to another two weeks and then another. It won't seem as overwhelming if you commit in bite-sized chunks. It may be a bit disruptive to start with but the benefits will quickly outweigh the initial inconvenience.

Nutrition basics

Put simply, food is broken down into two major areas: the macronutrients (carbohydrates, protein, fat, fibre); and the micronutrients (vitamins and minerals).

Carbohydrates

Carbohydrates are our main source of energy. They are absorbed into the body and become glucose which the body uses to run, jump, hop, play and think. Great sources of carbohydrates are fruit, vegetables, bread, cereals and pasta or any foods made with grains such as wheat, corn, rye, rice or barley. Some carbohydrates are broken down and utlised by the body soon after you eat them. These are said to have a high glycemic index or GI. Other carbohydrates have a more complex structure. They are broken down slowly and are utilised in a more sustained way and are rated low on the glycemic index. The best diet has a balance of both low GI and high GI foods, offering us a blend of both immediate and longer term energy.

Protein

Protein is used by our bodies for building everything from bones, muscle and tissue to blood and hormones. It comes in many shapes and sizes, from both animal and plant sources. A sedentary adult needs around 0.8 grams of protein per kilogram of body weight per day. This means a person weighing 70 kilograms needs about 56 grams per day. As a rough guide, an average-sized steak contains around 30 grams of protein, a 100-gram tin of tuna contains around 27 grams and an egg contains around 6 grams. So you can see that a couple of serves of lean protein per day will easily help you to meet your protein needs. Few of us have issues with getting enough protein. In fact, many of us eat too much.

Animal protein

Animal meat is called complete protein as it contains all of the protein building blocks that the body needs to get on with its business. Beef, veal, pork, ham, chicken, turkey, fish and other seafood, eggs, cheese, yoghurt and milk are all common sources of animal protein. Due to the saturated fat content of most animal protein, it is best to eat only lean sources of it.

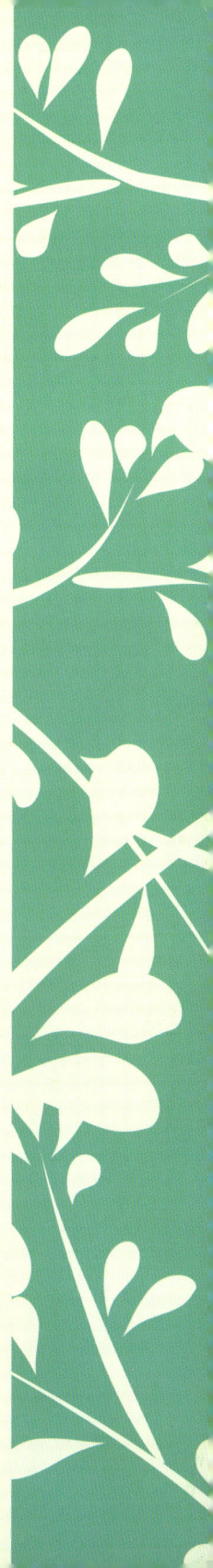

Plant protein

Common sources of plant protein include pulses, beans and legumes (soy beans, butter beans, cannellini beans, lentils, black-eyed peas, split peas, chickpeas, etc), all soy-bean products such as tofu or soy milk, nuts, seeds and also grains such as wheat, oats, barley, spelt, rice, kamut, triticale (a blend of wheat and rye), corn and rye. Plant protein does not have the saturated fats (the bad fats) that animal protein has and is a cornucopia of vitamins and minerals.

Although legumes, beans, grains, nuts and seeds are a very good source of protein, they are an incomplete protein, as each individual legume or bean variety does not contain all of the protein building blocks that the body needs. Some plants contain some of the blocks and other plants contain a different combination of blocks. To overcome this, combine different sources of plant protein into one meal. This sounds more difficult than it actually is.

Simple plant protein guidelines

Guideline 1: In the same meal have legume/pulse + grain

So that means things like…

Beans + wheat   Baked beans on wholemeal toast
Lentils + rice   Rice pasta with lentil pasta sauce
Chickpeas + corn   Hummus with corn crackers
Chickpeas + wheat   Chickpea flat bread
Kidney beans + corn   Corn pasta with kidney bean pasta sauce

Guideline 2: In the same meal have legume/pulse + nuts or seeds

So that means things like…

Chickpeas + sesame seeds   Hummus with sesame seeds
Tofu + almonds   Asian stir-fry with tofu and almonds
Tofu + ground seeds   Banana smoothie with tofu and ground
                                 seed mix

Fats

Fats naturally occur in food. We need them to live. Fat is calorie dense so it is a potent energy source. It is also vital for other functions such as helping us to absorb vitamins A, D, E and K. Fats are found in foods from animals (butter, cream, fat in meat) and plants (olive oil, avocado, nuts, seeds, coconut oil).

There are good and bad fats. The only difference between them is a small change in their chemical structure, but our bodies certainly notice the difference. 'Good' fats are the unsaturated ones called polyunsaturated and monounsaturated fats. 'Bad' fats are from animals, other than fish, and are called saturated fats. One other small class of fats is the trans fatty acids. Trans fats may be found in some commercial frying oils, fried foods, some margarines, shop-bought bakery items and some highly processed foods. Nutrition labels with hydrogenated or partially hydrogenated oils listed in their ingredients contain trans fats. Most full-fat dairy products, beef and sheep products contain naturally produced trace amounts of trans fatty acids.

Separating the fat from the fiction

The Fat	The Effect	The Food*
Saturated fats and trans fatty acids	Too much of these is not good for long-term health	Animal meat, cream, butter, coconut cream, palm oil, snack foods and fast foods with hydrogenated oil listed on their nutrition panel.
Unsaturated fat: monounsaturated	Positive effect on health	Olives, ground nut oils, avocados.
Unsaturated fat: polyunsaturated	Positive effect on health	Sunflower seeds, flaxseed oil, walnuts and oily fish such as salmon, sardines and mackerel.

*The foods listed are examples of where these fats can be found. There are many more sources in addition to these examples.

Bad fats can cause damage to our cells, give our heart and blood vessels a hard time and make us more vulnerable to disease. Most people eat about 20% more than the recommended maximum amount of saturated fat. The average man should have no more than 24 grams of saturated fat a day and the average woman no more than 20 grams of saturated fat a day. To put this into perspective, a large burger from a popular fast food chain contains 10.6 grams of saturated fat, nearly half the recommended total daily intake for a woman. If you want to reduce your saturated fat intake, have a look at the 21 Day Sat Fat Challenge at www.eatwell.gov.uk/healthydiet/fss/fats/satfat.

To move the balance from the bad fats to the good fats in your diet, try using a good quality spread made from canola, sunflower, olive or sesame oil instead of butter. Also eat oily fish such as mackerel, sardines or salmon twice a week. Use monounsaturated or polyunsaturated cooking oils such as olive, sunflower or sesame instead of butter or ghee, and use baking recipes that stipulate oil instead of butter.

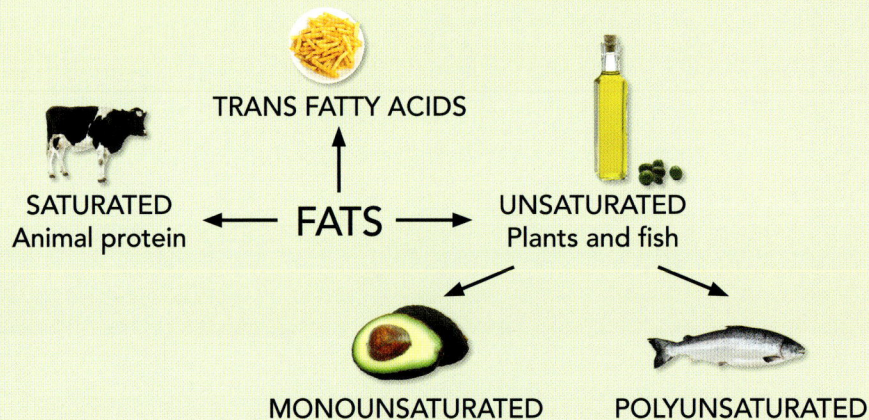

TRANS FATTY ACIDS

SATURATED
Animal protein

FATS

UNSATURATED
Plants and fish

MONOUNSATURATED

POLYUNSATURATED

Fibre

Fibre is essential in every person's diet. It helps to maintain a healthy digestive tract, keep your bowels regular and slows the release of food sugar or glucose into the blood.

There are three types of fibre: insoluble, soluble and resistant starch. Insoluble fibre is found in some grains such as wheat and wheat bran. Soluble fibre is the fibre found in fruit and vegetables and grains such as oats. Resistant starch is abundant in wholegrains (such as those found in cold wholemeal pasta or brown rice) and legumes.

By ensuring you have enough soluble fibre in your diet you will be helping to reduce the risk of developing many serious diseases such as heart disease and bowel cancer in later life. Bowel cancer is still the second most common cancer in Australia, so most of us would greatly benefit from an increase in fibre in our diets.

Great sources of fibre include dried fruit, apples, pears, sweet potatoes, wholemeal bread, oats, brown rice and carrots. For more information on fibre and how to easily meet your fibre needs, check out 'Fibre friendly – easy ways to boost your fibre' on page 52.

Five golden rules to keep your engines firing on all cylinders

Fresh is best

The fresher the fruit, vegetables and meat that you eat, the richer the food will be in vitamins, minerals and other nutritional goodies. Organic food is an excellent choice as often the taste is better, the nutrients are more plentiful and there are no pesticides, hormones or antibiotics. If you cannot afford or find good fresh organic produce, ensure the conventional produce you buy is as fresh as possible.

Use food that's as close to it's natural state as possible, that is, whole food

The 'natural state' means food that is as unprocessed as possible. Processing alters the perfectly designed nutritional package that nature intended for us and so degrades the nutrition of foods and the benefits that they offer our bodies. An example of nature's design brilliance can be seen in many iron-rich foods, for example dried apricots are rich in vitamin C, which is the very vitamin that we need to readily absorb iron!

Unfortunately, when foods are processed, it is often the helpers such as vitamin C that are lost and so the nutritional benefit of the food is diminished. So use wholemeal and wholegrain foods (wholemeal flour and pasta, brown rice, etc.). If you don't like the wholegrain stuff, try a slow introduction by mixing them into your current processed foods. Over time, increase the ratio of the whole food and phase out the processed food. Wholemeal and wholegrain foods do need to be cooked longer than their processed counterparts, if they are not, they will be tough, fibrous and unappetising. For example white rice may take 20 minutes, but brown rice will need at least 30 minutes to become soft and fluffy.

Variety is key

Variety is an essential element to a great diet. Nature has planned our food beautifully, making some foods rich in particular vitamins and minerals and others rich in different, often complementary, vitamins and minerals. So eat a diet that is varied in order to get a little bit of all the good things you need.

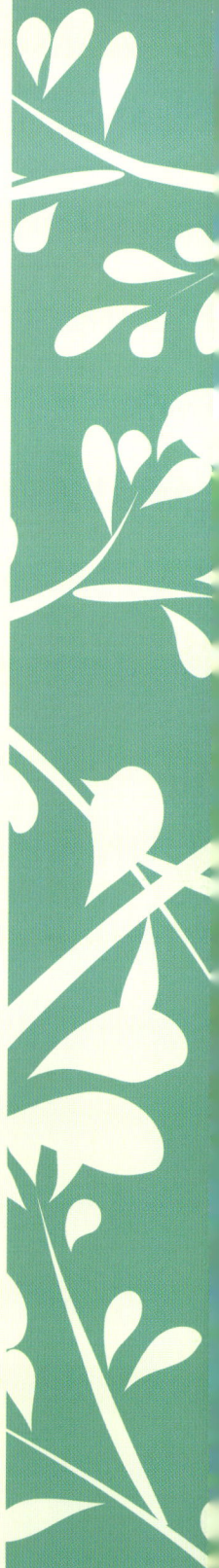

There are some easy ways to ensure you get variety in your diet. For foods like fruit and vegetables, their colours often indicate their different nutritional strengths. For example, red foods (such as capsicum and tomato) are generally very high in vitamin C and lycopene; green foods (such as spinach and broccoli) are high in vitamins A, C, E, cholorphyll and iron; orange and yellow foods (such as carrots and citrus fruits) are high in vitamin A; dark blue and purple foods (such as grapes and eggplant) are high in vitamin C; and white foods (such as garlic and onion) are high in organo sulphides which can help keep cold and flu bugs away. So, across the week, try to include as many colours in your diet as possible.

Get out of your comfort zone and try some new foods. Try one new vegetable each week for a month or at the beginning of a new season when all of the new seasonal bounty arrives in the shop. Pick up some celeriac or kohlrabi, perhaps slow roast a turnip or make some parsnip oven chips, or maybe even try some choko? Okay, maybe not the choko...

Keep the balance right

For the average sedentary adult, around half the average 25-centimetre dinner plate should be filled with vegetables or salad, one quarter filled with carbohydrates and one quarter with protein such as meat, legumes, chicken. If you are trying to lose weight, then two thirds of your plate should be plant food like vegetables and salad.

Manage the baddies

Inherent in this whole food recommendation is the idea that over time sugar and salt need to be minimised, all artificial colours and flavours need to be removed, and your good fats need to be boosted while reducing your bad saturated and trans fats. Eating sugar, salt and artificial colours and flavours in large quantities only depletes your body of vitamins and minerals. Sugar and salt occur naturally in foods, but not in the vast quantities or refined form in which we eat them. In fact, 75% of the salt we eat is already in the processed food we buy, making label checking even more important if you are trying to tone up your diet.

The most important nutrients

This chapter would not be complete without a discussion of some of the most important nutrients we need to keep us powering along. The following table is included to give you a quick reference to the vital nutrients, why they are vital and where they can be found in abundance.

Important nutrients, some of their major roles and great food sources

Nutrient	Major roles	Great sources
Vitamin A	Is an antioxidant. Role in hormone synthesis, bone growth, increases resistance to infection, skin health.	Apricots, carrots, green leafy vegetables, broccoli, sweet potato, tomatoes, rockmelon.
Bioflavinoids	Is an antioxidant. Protects vitamin C.	Buckwheat, citrus fruits, skin of fruit and vegetables.
Vitamin B group	Energy production and numerous other vital body functions, including digestion, growth and blood-sugar regulation.	Legumes, wheat germ, whole grains, avocado, eggs, broccoli, almonds, chicken, meat, green vegetables, mushrooms, sardines.
Folic acid	Nerve and blood health.	Green leafy vegetables, lentils, eggs.
Vitamin C	Is an antioxidant. Role in bone and teeth health, immunity, improves iron absorption.	Broccoli, citrus fruits, peas, cabbage, kiwi, guava, sweet potato, berries, strawberries.
Vitamin D	Helps calcium absorption and bone health; supports immunity.	Eggs, sunflower seeds, alfalfa sprouts, milk, sardines, tuna, sunlight.
Vitamin E	Is an antioxidant and anti-inflammatory; supports immunity.	Almonds, beef, corn, eggs, rye, oats, nuts, wheat germ.
Essential fatty acids	Heart and nerve health; anti-inflammatory.	Pepitas, linseed oil, sunflower seeds, nuts, deep-sea fish, avocado.
Calcium	Bone, heart, nerve and muscle health; blood-sugar regulation.	Almonds, broccoli, buckwheat, dairy, figs, egg yolk, green leafy vegetables.
Iodine	Healthy thyroid function.	Mushrooms, oysters, sunflower seeds.
Iron	Supports immunity; used in making red blood cells and delivering oxygen; role in skin and nail formation.	Apricots, parsley, red meat, sunflower seeds, pepitas, egg yolk, chicken, green vegetables.
Magnesium	Heart, muscle, bone and nerve health.	Wheat germ, cashews, Brazil nuts, parsnip, sesame seeds, walnuts, eggs.
Zinc	Supports immunity; role in healing and skin.	Cashews, beef, egg yolk, milk, sunflower seeds, pepitas, whole grains, rice.

Back in the real world: RDIs vs RDOs

So the nutritional theory is great, but what about back in the real world? You've just gotten home from work, your partner is not home until 8pm, the dog has fleas, the kids are tearing each other's hair out and you've got nothing in the fridge.

Take heart, a bit of planning and balance will keep you on track, whether you are living alone or are the head of a Brady Bunch. The aim is to eat well 80% of the time, to meet your RDIs (recommended daily intakes) by packing your diet with lean protein and fresh fruit and vegetables but 20% of the time, take an RDO (rostered day off), put your feet up and treat yourself. Life is about feeling great and part of feeling great is taking pleasure in eating, relaxing and giving yourself a rest from it all.

RDIs

Planning is the key to making eating well easy. Take 20 minutes on a Sunday evening to jot down a menu plan for the week, then do a shopping list. 'What's for dinner?' takes a lot of daily headspace, so a 20-minute investment in planning resolves that daily worry and gives you a much greater chance of sticking to your healthy eating plan. If you have it ready and waiting in the fridge each night, a healthy dinner is easy. Try to keep the weekend meals easy to prepare and fun, to give you minimal time in the kitchen.

Monday	Sweet chilli stir-fried vegetables with egg
Tuesday	Minestrone
Wednesday	Beef shaslicks with orange mash and a green salad
Thursday	Thai fish cakes with Greek salad and salsa
Friday	Hamburgers with the lot
Saturday	Homemade Hawaiian pizzas with rainbow salad
Sunday	Vegetable curry (homemade from the freezer)

RDOs

Have an RDO each fortnight – don't go crazy, but give yourself a break. This will satisfy your cravings and also help you to stick to your plan for the rest of the time. If you are looking to lose weight, save your RDOs until you reach a weight loss goal and then let yourself have a *small* indulgence. The most common indulgence I see in my clinic is chocolate. It must be the single most craved food in the Western world! If you are a chocoholic, have a few squares of good quality dark chocolate on your RDO, but then put the block away as you don't want to undo all of your hard work in one fell swoop.

Meeting your 2&5

The recommended daily intake of fruit and vegetables is two serves of fruit and five of vegetables. To check if you are getting your 2&5 you can use the 'How Am I Doing?' quiz at www.gofor2and5.com.au.

Examples of a serve of vegetables	Examples of a serve of fruit

½ cup cooked vegetables
1 medium potato
1 cup salad vegetables
½ cup cooked legumes
   (dried beans, peas or lentils)
	150g fresh fruit which equals
	   1 medium-sized piece (eg apple)
	   or 2 smaller pieces (eg apricots)
	1 cup canned or chopped fruit
	½ cup (125ml) 100% fruit juice
	1½ tablespoons dried fruit
	   (eg sultanas or 4 dried apricot halves)
	(www.gofor2and5.com.au)

Below are some easy, painless ways to cheat your way to 2&5 by packing all of it into one meal.

- A jacket potato with 1 cup baked beans and 2 cups side salad followed by an apple and 4 dried apricots = 2&5

- Vegetable omelette with ½ cup grated pumpkin and zucchini, 1 cup coleslaw with pineapple, an orange to finish and a virgin bloody Mary to sip = 2&5

- A fresh juice with 3 carrots, a celery stalk, some beetroot, 2 apples and 2 oranges = 2&5

- 1½ cups leftover mashed vegetables and baked beans on toast with a glass of fresh orange juice = 2&5

- Cajun chicken with 2 cups stir-fried carrots, broccoli, cabbage, capsicum and onion followed by a banana and strawberry smoothie for dessert = 2&5

Healthy Eating Snapshot

	What they are	What we need	What they do
Carbohydrates	Simple carbs	Less of these	High GI, short-term energy burst, blood-sugar spike
	Complex carbs	More of these	Low GI, longer term energy, more stable blood sugar
Protein	Animal protein	Less of this	Complete protein but high in saturated fat
	Plant protein	More of this	Incomplete protein (so combine a couple of sources), low in fat and high in nutrients and fibre
Fats	Bad fats	Less of these	Saturated and trans fats are lazy fats if we consume too much of them. They can clog arteries and cause health problems
	Good fats	More of these	Monounsaturated and polyunsaturated such as Omega 3. This is a good fat, great for general health and reducing the risk of many degenerative diseases
Fibre	Soluble fibre	More of this	Helps lower blood cholesterol
	Insoluble fibre & resistant starch	More of this	Excellent for bowel health

This snapshot is included as a general guide only for a healthy meat eater. Individual health factors such as diabetes need to be taken into consideration. Please consult your healthcare professional before making any major changes to your diet.

What is fat? What is fab?

Fat is not the only way to determine if a recipe needs a makeover. The pre-makeover 'fat' recipes in this book are often high in fat, salt, sugar, low in fibre, devoid of nutrients and are sometimes even thrown into the deep fryer. They are nutritionally lacking and so I call them fat recipes.

Next time you scan your cookbooks looking for dinner ideas, use this quick checklist to see which are the fat recipes.

The Fat Checklist

Check for a nutritional panel at the bottom of the recipe.

If the fat is over 20 grams of fat per serve, it is a high-fat recipe. Take particular note of the saturated fat which should be listed under the total fat. Once you start checking these, you will be surprised. Some curries and creamy dishes contain over 65 grams of fat and 20 grams of saturated fat! If the sugar is over 15 grams per 100-gram serve, the recipe is high in sugar. If the sodium is over 120 milligrams per 100 gram serve, it is high in salt. If all of these are over the limit, it is a heart attack on a plate! If you are really keen, you can use an online recipe calculator to see how much fat is in your homemade recipes.

1. Scan for high-saturated fat ingredients
If there is no nutritional panel, cast your eye over the recipe and look for any of these ingredients: butter, coconut milk, full-cream milk, cream, ice-cream, hard cheeses, mascarpone, crème fraîche, streaky bacon, 2 egg yolks per serve, processed meats, gravies, pastry, cheap or fatty cuts of meat and butter-based sauces such as hollandaise. If that reads like a list of your favourite foods, don't worry, have a look at 'Fat lot of good' on page 92 for smart ways to cut the fat.

2. Scan for processed foods
This includes white rice, pasta and flour, all of which are devoid of fibre.

3. Scan for high salt or sugar
In a recipe, this means anything more than a pinch of salt or in a sweet dish more than ¾ cup (165g) of sugar, depending on the dish size and the number of serves.

4. Scan for nutrient dense foods

How many different fruit or vegetables are in the dish?

5. Check out the quality of the protein

The protein needs to be lean if it is animal protein. Chuck steak, osso bucco and any other cheap, fatty cuts of meat are filled with saturated fat. Any plant protein content is fantastic.

6. Take note of the cooking method

Even the healthiest meal in the world would lose all of its points if it were cooked in the deep fryer or boiled for an hour and drained. The cooking method can make or break a potentially fab recipe. It can add fat and kill nutrients. For example, a crumbed and fried chicken schnitzel can contain as much as six times the amount of fat as a grilled skinless chicken breast. This doesn't mean that everything has to be grilled. Find some middle ground such as crumbing then baking.

If your recipe flies through the Fat Checklist, then you have a fab recipe, so start cooking. If it failed one or two, do your own makeover. You don't need to make over every aspect of the recipe. You could just make over an area each time you use the recipe. Making one change at a time may help to slowly retrain your tastebuds and also maintain the support of your family or partner.

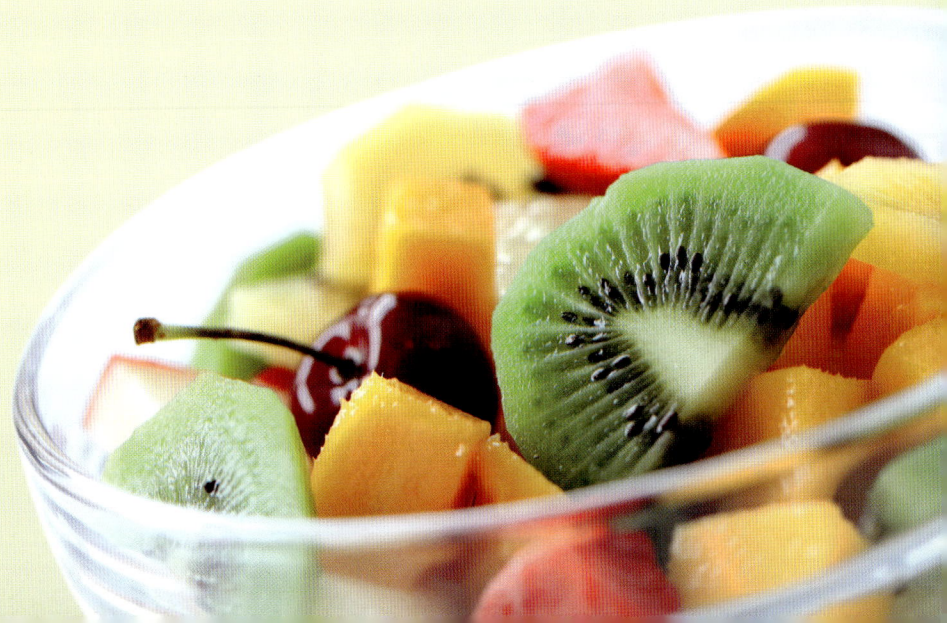

The Fab Makeover
Sugar makeover

Sugar is so refined, it is devoid of all of its original nutrients and, to be absorbed, it actually robs our body of nutrients. Reducing sugar doesn't mean using artificial sweeteners. Sugar is a completely natural product and regardless of contributing no nutrients to our diet, it is superior to artificial sweeteners. Reducing sugar means, first, replacing it with other natural, more nutritious sweeteners and, second, reducing the level of sweetness you have become accustomed to. Here are lots of ideas for doing a sugar makeover in your kitchen.

- When sweetening foods, such as cereals and drinks, use less processed sweeteners such as pure maple syrup, agave syrup, barley malt syrup or apple and pear juice concentrate.

- In baking, an amount of sugar is vital for flavour, bulk, structure, browning, aroma and to help the cakes and biscuits retain moisture, so we can minimise it but not leave it out. Never reduce the sugar by more than one half of the amount stated in the original recipe or you will change the chemistry of the cake and could end up with a flop. In most recipes (except jams, meringues or ice-cream), the sugar can be halved with no disastrous results or you can experiment with other natural sweeteners.

- Rather than icing a cake, buy a ready-made shaker filled with icing sugar or fill your own shaker and sprinkle the cake with the icing sugar just before serving. If you want to be fancy, place a paper doyley on top of the cake and then shake over the icing sugar. Carefully remove the doyley and you have a pattern on the cake. It looks pretty and dresses the cake but uses less than a tablespoon of sugar, whereas icing the entire cake would use up to a full cup of icing sugar.

- Use dried or fresh fruit puree to replace the sugar in some baking recipes. This works well in some biscuit recipes, breads and brownies. It reduces fat, boosts nutrients and fibre and allows you to cut down on added sugar without compromising sweetness. Make a thick fruit puree using dried fruit and a small amount of water or fresh fruit on its own. Substitute the same weight of the puree for all or some of the sugar in the recipe. Experiment to get the texture you want.

- Always use very ripe fruit which is rich in natural sugars so you don't need to add any extra sweetness. When using tinned fruit in your recipes, use fruit tinned in juice not syrup.

- In savoury and unbaked desserts, sugar is not as vital and can be reduced to an amount that your tastebuds will tolerate.

Fat makeover

Fat and salt are core flavour ingredients in many recipes and need to be carefully tailored in your makeover so that you don't end up with a healthy, flavourless blob.

- Where possible, reduce or omit high fat ingredients. Replace mayonnaise with a creamy dressing made with yoghurt or buttermilk, serve nachos without the sour cream, leave out the bacon or use rindless and 97% fat-free bacon and serve your desserts with gelato instead of full-fat ice-cream.

- Butter can be replaced by lower fat monounsaturated spreads (such as those made from seed oils) but if you bake with a spread that has a fat content lower than 40%, you may need to experiment a little before you get perfect results.

- Replace sour cream with low-fat natural yoghurt or use a reduced amount of extra low-fat or no-fat sour cream in sauces and casseroles. Yoghurt has the same natural tartness as sour cream without the fat. Add it to your cooking just before serving (it will separate if it is allowed to boil) or mix it with a small amount of cornflour before adding it to the dish to help stabilise it and reduce the chance of curdling.

- When mashing vegetables, replace cream and butter with low-fat milk or yoghurt and reduced-salt stock. If you use half skim milk and half stock, you get a creamy, tasty mash without the fat.

- Allow soups and stocks to cool then skim the fat off. This can skim off up to 400 kilojoules per tablespoon.

- Use lean cuts of meat such as 97% fat-free bacon, lean steak instead of chuck steak or chicken breast instead of leg (yes this means throwing out the very tasty chicken skin). Removing the fat from steak before you cook it can reduce the fat by up to half. Generally, the more white you see on meat, the more fat it contains. For pre-packaged meat, you can compare the fat content on the nutritional labels to find the best option.

- Use low-fat versions of dairy when you can. For milk and yoghurt this means less than 1.5 grams of fat per 100 grams. All cakes, pancakes and other batters can be made with skim, low-fat milk or buttermilk. Buttermilk tastes rich and creamy but is actually low in fat, is filled with lots of nutrients and is great for digestion. Its acidity works during the cooking process to make your cakes and batters fluffier than normal milk. It is also great for making low-fat creamy salad dressings. In baking, you will get better results with semi-skim (1.6% fat) or evaporated skim milk rather than full skim (0.5% fat) milk, as some of the fat in the milk improves the outcome of the baked goods. Keep full skim milk for custards, mashes and sauces.

• When you need whipped cream, replace the cream with chilled low-fat evaporated milk. Use it immediately after whipping. Even the full-fat evaporated milk contains 75% less fat than cream.

• When serving desserts, opt for one of the fab creams on pages 216–217 or a low-fat ice-cream (less than 5% fat). Choose an ice-cream with a short ingredients list that is easy to pronounce and understand, that is, an ice-cream made from real food not in a chemistry lab. You'll quickly see which brands are more committed to natural ingredients than others.

• Cheeses vary greatly in their fat content. Choose cheese with less than 10 grams of fat per 100 grams. This means the white, un-aged cheeses such as low-fat cottage cheese, ricotta, quark and Indian paneer cheese. Use low-fat and salt-reduced fetta or goat's cheese in salads, on pizzas, in pasta sauces and in sandwiches. Try low-fat mozzarella on pizzas and in toasted sandwiches for a lovely stringy finish. Use a blend of low-fat cream cheese and sieved low-fat cottage cheese in your cheesecakes and you will notice no difference in taste or texture. Refer to 'A closer look at cheese' on page 245 in Resources for more information on the nutritional content of cheeses.

• Cut out cheese from sauces. Instead, sprinkle a small amount on top of the served dish and allow it to melt. The cheese will be the first thing you taste, giving you that lovely cheesy flavour with a minimum amount of fat and salt.

• Find a recipe that uses good quality oil instead of butter. The oils are still high in fat but the fat is unsaturated. When using oil in your recipes, ensure it is good quality oil such as extra virgin olive oil or a nut oil. If you use a vegetable oil, ensure it is labelled as unsaturated. If it is not, it is highly likely to be saturated palm oil. Butter-free or low-fat cakes and other baked goods may not keep as long as the full-fat versions as the fat helps to retain the cake's moisture.

• In recipes such as shortbread, curds, rich fruit cakes, traditional pastry and some preserves, low-fat spreads and oil cannot be substituted as the chemistry of the recipe depends too heavily on the fat from the butter. Avoid these recipes or only use them occasionally.

- Use a spray oil or measure out your oil before you put it in the heated pan and it will help to reduce the amount of oil you use for your cooking.

- Choose spreads or oils that have a nut or seed oil listed as their first ingredient.

- If using pastry, use a 25% reduced-fat pastry or use filo pastry and use spray oil between each filo layer rather than brushing with butter.

- If making a creamy curry, use coconut flavoured low-fat evaporated milk. It has 92% less fat than regular coconut milk and 95% less fat than cream but tastes just as delicious.

- Make salad dressings with little or no oil, such as the Dijon mustard dressing on page 166 or the Caesar salad dressing on page 70. Keep a couple of empty glass jam jars and make two or three salad dressings to keep in the fridge. Label them clearly and they will always be conveniently on hand to dress a salad and reduce the risk of you reaching for the egg mayonnaise or thousand island.

- When baking, choose your recipes carefully. Some cakes are naturally low in fat, needing no makeover and so you are guaranteed a great result. Naturally high-fat cakes are shortened cakes like butter cakes and pound cakes. Naturally low-fat cakes are foam cakes. No-fat foam cakes are angel food cakes, dacquoises and meringues. Foam cakes with fat from egg yolks only are sponge cakes and roulades, and foam cakes with fat from egg yolks *and* shortening (like butter or oil) are genoises and chiffon cakes. Look for foam cake recipes when choosing a cake recipe and choose those that are also lower in sugar. If you are altering baking recipes, it can help to add an extra ½ teaspoon of baking powder to give the cake an added lift. When you are greasing the tins, substitute spray oil for butter and line them with baking paper to reduce the amount of fat absorbed by the cakes, muffins or breads.

- The fat in eggs is in the yolks, so if you are watching your weight use only the whites where possible. They are fat free, are filled with nutrients and possess the raising ability we need in cakes and other baking. If you are not watching your weight, keep the whole egg in the recipe as there is great nutrition in a whole egg.

- Don't buy ingredients soaking in oil. For example, instead of sun-dried tomatoes, buy dried tomatoes and soak them in some warm water for 10–15 minutes to reconstitute them. The problem with buying them in oil is not only the fat content, it is also the poor quality of the oil many products soak in.

Fibre makeover

Unfortunately, high fibre foods are not popular. Many people find them too chewy or bulky, as they are accustomed to the white processed foods that do not need to be well chewed. If you cook wholemeal and wholegrain products well and make the transition slowly, your body will love you for it and your tastebuds will adapt and learn to love the taste of the whole food.

• Use wholemeal flour and wholegrains in your cooking.

• Add a cup of soup mix, pearl barley or split peas to your soups and casseroles.

• Mash white beans, such as butter beans or cannellini beans, and add to your potato or mixed vegetable mashes.

• Add some kidney beans or raw red lentils to your pasta sauces.

• To boost the fibre content of your dishes, sprinkle some psyllium over your breakfast cereal or pop some in a milkshake or smoothie.

• Try any of the nutrient makeover ideas below, as fruit and vegetables are a wonderful source of fibre.

Salt makeover

Salt upsets your kidneys and, long term, can affect the way your cardiovascular system operates. There are lots of ways to reduce salt in your recipes and cooking.

• Herbs, spices, lemon juice and vinegars are the best way to reduce salt without cutting out flavour. See 'Quick guide to using herbs and spices' on page 239 in Resources for a list of the many ways to use different herbs and spices. It's a great idea to grow your favourites as they are at their most flavoursome when just picked and you can pick as you need rather than having to buy a whole bunch at a time. They are also very easy to grow. See the kitchen garden list on page 35 for a list of the best and easiest herbs to grow.

• Don't add salt to the water when cooking pasta or vegetables.

• Give your tastebuds time to retrain to low-salt foods. It will take a while, but you will begin to notice the other flavours within the food.

• Use foods as fresh as possible. This means that not only will their nutrients be maximised, so will their natural flavour.

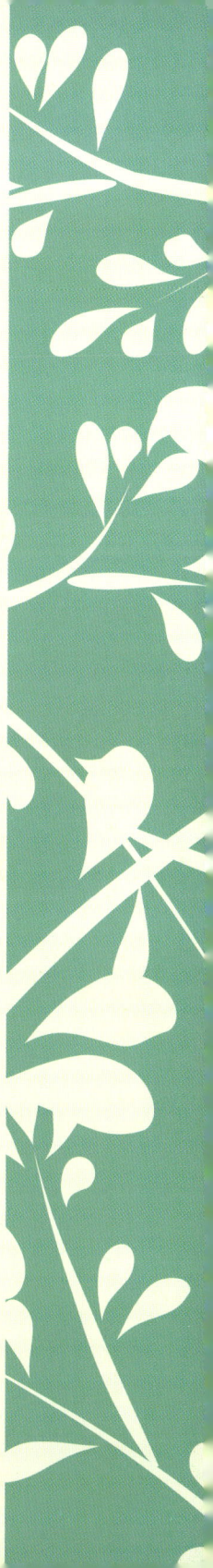

- Buy and cook with foods labelled as low salt or no added salt.

- Never add more than a pinch of salt and only if your dish really needs it. As you will see from the recipes in this book, some recipes do need a pinch of salt and this is fine. This means in the total dish, not per serve. Putting this into perspective, if you were to buy a pre-prepared bolognese pasta meal from a shop, the sodium content would be around 562 milligrams per serve (that is, around ¼ teaspoon of salt per serve). A pinch of salt is approximately ⅛ of a teaspoon and in your homemade bolognese dish, this ⅛ teaspoon is being divided into eight serves, which would make the salt intake per person minimal. It is certainly important not to have salt on the table or add it liberally to everything, but at times, a very small amount is needed.

Nutrient makeover

The best way to give recipes a nutrient makeover is to add fruit and vegetables or easily incorporated foods like nutrient-dense wheat germ or legumes.

- Boost the vegetables in all of your stir-fries, stews, salads, soups and casseroles while reducing the meat. It's cheaper and more nutritious and a great way to make your vegetables tastier if you are not a big fan of plain steamed vegetables.

- Add fruit to your dessert recipes. It may mean serving it on the side or actually incorporating it into the recipe. Opt for an apple cake or carrot cake instead of a plain butter cake.

- Add a 400-gram tin of legumes (chickpeas, butter beans, kidney beans) or some red lentils to your soups, stews and casseroles.

- Add a couple of tablespoons of wheat germ to your cake and bread recipes or throw it into your smoothies.

- Add a shop-bought bottle or pack of vegetable juice to your sauces, casseroles, soups and stews. Buy brands that are 100% juice and contain little or no added salt or sugar.

- Cook up extra dinner vegetables, then puree them and freeze them in ice-cube trays. Place them in snaplock bags in the freezer. When you need to thicken a sauce, casserole or stew, add some of the pureed vegetables.

- Keep some shop-bought frozen vegetables in the freezer for those days when you have not had time to get to the shops. Although the taste does not compare with fresh vegetables, frozen vegetables can still be very high in some essential nutrients.

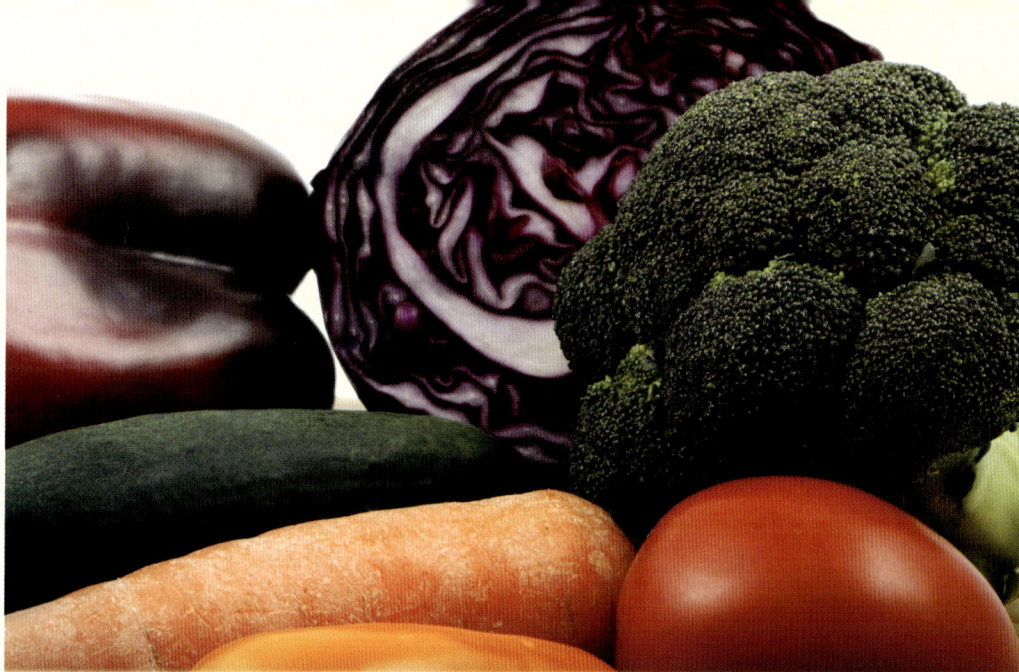

- If you find vegetables boring, try serving your main dish with a vegetable packed sauce that carries some spice. Try a ratatouille (page 178) or a fresh salsa (pages 164 and 165). These sides are packed with vegetables and their lovely spicy flavours make you forget they contain any veggies at all.

Protein makeover

The makeover goal for protein is to reduce the amount of saturated fat (that is, fat from animal meats and products) and also to boost the variety of protein.

- Reduce the animal protein in your recipes by bumping up the vegetables.

- Use plant protein like peas and other legumes. They are cheap, easy to use and don't contain saturated fat.

- When using meat, trim excess fat and remove all skin. Marinade or sear it to seal in the flavour and moisture if you are using it in a casserole as lean cuts can sometimes dry out when cooked for prolonged periods.

- Don't put stuffing inside the roasting meat as it absorbs a lot of the fat melting from the cooking meat. Cook your stuffing separately.

- If you can, cool your casseroles, soups or stews before serving so that you can skim off any excess fat.

Cooking method makeover

The best cooking methods are those that enhance the flavour of the food, don't add any nasties and don't take away any goodies.

- The best way to makeover your cooking method is to put the deep-fryer at the back of the cupboard and keep it there.

- Grilling, steaming, baking, poaching, stir-frying in minimal oil or cooking in a non-stick frying pan are the best cooking methods. If your recipe calls for frying, try instead spraying the food lightly with some olive oil and grill it or bake it in an oven on 220°C to get a crispy finish. If it says to boil vegetables or fruit, steam them instead to retain nutrients.

- When stir-frying, add a tablespoon of extra virgin olive oil to the heated pan, throw the raw ingredients in and toss for a couple of minutes, then add a small amount of water and place the lid on for another couple of minutes. This allows the vegetables to steam and reduces the temperature of the oil slightly so that it does not reach smoking point which can alter its chemical structure and become slightly toxic.

- Roast meat on a rack in a roasting tin so the fat can run off.

- If you do roast or lightly fry food, always place the cooked food on absorbent kitchen paper to drain any excess fat.

- Cook food only until it is a golden yellow not brown, and never eat burnt food (including burnt toast), which is high in acrymalides and which studies have shown increases the risk of some cancers.

- When barbecuing or browning chicken or meat, reduce the amount of carcinogenic nasties produced by marinating the meat in a marinade containing some sugar (for example, soy and honey, sweet chilli or honey, ginger and orange). Even marinating for as little as five minutes can help to reduce the number of nasty chemicals formed by the barbecuing and browning process.

The Fab Kitchen

With only one or two exceptions, this book uses everyday equipment and items that are readily available in most homes. All of the major food items are listed below.

Remember, to keep the pantry and fridge well-stocked with delicious, healthy fresh vegetables and fruit. These foods are the key to achieving healthy eating habits and being able to quickly whip up some fab meals, thereby easily resisting the urge to resort to the traditional fat meals or high fat takeaways.

Equipment

Absorbent kitchen paper
Baking dish, 1 litre ovenproof
Baking paper, non-stick
Baking trays, non-stick
Cake tins, various shapes and sizes, non-stick
Food processor and/or hand blender
Frying pan, non-stick
Grater, good quality
Griddle pan, non-stick
Jars, glass, small and large
Knives, a set of good quality sharp knives
Muffin pan, 12-hole
Pastry brush, bristle
Saucepans, good quality, heavy-based
Scales, digital
Sieve
Slotted spoon
Wok, non-stick
Zester

The pantry

Staples

Baking powder
Bicarbonate of soda (baking soda)
Bread: wholemeal, soy and linseed or rye bread or fortified, high-fibre white
Breadcrumbs, wholemeal if possible
Chocolate melts, white and milk
Cocoa powder, unsweetened (check the label to ensure no sugar has been added)
Cooking spray: canola or olive oil
Corn crackers
Cornflour
Cornmeal
Dates
Desiccated coconut
Flour: self-raising white and wholemeal, and plain white and wholemeal
Garlic
Gelatine, powdered
Golden syrup
Icing sugar

Legumes, tinned, such as chickpeas, kidney beans and four bean mix (no added salt)

Lemons

Maple syrup, pure

Milk, evaporated full-fat, skim milk, and coconut-flavoured milk

Noodles: Singapore and rice

Oil (monounsaturated), such as peanut oil, sesame oil, extra virgin olive oil and good quality vegetable oil (not derived from palm oil)

Onion

Pasta (preferably wholegrain): lasagne and fettuccine

Pineapple juice

Poppy seeds

Red lentils

Rice: preferably brown and basmati

Rolled oats

Rum extract

Salsa, low-salt

Skim milk powder

Sponge finger biscuits

Sugar: raw, brown and caster sugar

Sultanas

Tomatoes, tinned and diced

Tuna, tinned in spring water

Vanilla: natural vanilla paste or essence

Flavourings and condiments

Balsamic, white wine and white vinegar

Dijon and wholegrain mustard

Herbs and spices: the most commonly used dried herbs and spices are allspice, bay leaves, cayenne pepper, chilli flakes, cinnamon, cloves, coriander, cumin, curry powder, garlic powder, ginger powder, mixed herbs, mustard powder, nutmeg, onion powder, oregano, paprika, thyme and turmeric.

Pepper, white and black

Sauces: barbecue, fish, hoisin, low-salt soy, light soy, oyster, sweet chilli, Tabasco, tamari, tomato and Worcestershire. (Check labels carefully to make sure that all sauces are low in salt and contain no artificial ingredients.)

Sea salt

Sherry, dry (the alcohol will evaporate when cooked)

Tomato chutney or relish, good quality

Tomato paste

Vegetable stock, low-salt beef stock, low-salt chicken stock

The fridge

Bacon, 97% fat-free

Buttermilk (can be frozen until needed)

Cheese: low-fat cottage, ricotta or bocconcini; low-fat tasty Cheddar; 80% reduced-fat cream cheese; and parmesan

Curry pastes, green and red (check the labels carefully for fat content which varies considerably between brands)

Eggs, free-range

Milk, low-fat or skim

Soda water

Spread, low-fat based on nut or seed oils

Yoghurt, low-fat natural or low-fat Greek

Wheat germ

The freezer

Beef, organic low-fat minced

Berries, frozen, mixed (some cheaper brands use strawberries in their mixed berries. Avoid these as they are too large for baking and only useful when you are pureeing the berries)

Chicken breast fillets, skinless and free-range

Filo pastry

Ice-cream, low-fat vanilla

Kaffir lime leaves (freeze in a snaplock bag)

Lebanese bread

Lemon sorbet

Mozzarella cheese, grated low-fat

Puff pastry, 25% reduced-fat

Shortcrust pastry, 25% reduced-fat

The kitchen garden

Baby spinach

Basil, sweet and Thai

Dill

Mint, ordinary and Vietnamese

Oregano

Parsley

Rosemary

Salad: rocket, mizuna and mixed salad greens

Thyme

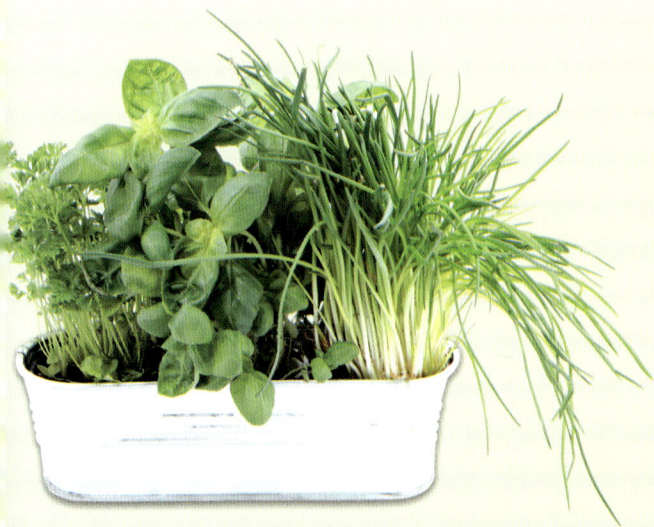

Going a step further

Some of you may be very happy with the fab lemon meringue pie, pizza and lasagne. Others of you may be looking to upgrade your diet in a bigger way so it has a lasting effect on your health and the changes become part of your everyday eating plan. If that's what you are looking to do, then this chapter is for you.

Life often gets in the way of our best intentions, and plans are slowly abandoned under the pressure of everyday chaos. A bit of forward planning can make a huge difference to your ability to give your diet a makeover.

Before embarking on your noble venture, choose how far you want to go. You may choose a premium economy diet and only change a few things here and there, or maybe a business-class diet with a few major permanent changes, or better still a first-class diet which gives you a major overhaul. Even if you are already on a first-class diet, you can still do some things to fine tune it further. Whatever class you are looking to sit in, the steps to get there will be the same.

Let's cut it down into bite-sized chunks, or five fat to fab steps, that can help you set yourself up for a healthy diet makeover.

Step 1. Set goals and rewards

Set yourself or your family small achievable goals. This gives you clear aims and will help to keep you motivated. It also gives you and everyone else in the family a clear plan of what the focus is for the week. If you are looking to achieve a specific goal, then your weekly goals need to build towards that goal. For example, a person looking to lose weight might reduce their portion size in week one and then work on limiting snacking. Making the changes one at a time will help you to incorporate them into your everyday routine and so increase the chances of them becoming a permanent change.

The note on the right is an example of weekly goals for a person looking to improve their general health and wellbeing.

Healthy eating goals

Week 1: Eat at least 5 different vegetables daily.

Week 2: Drink 2 litres of water each day.

Week 3: Try 5 new foods this week.

Week 4: Eat 3 different fruits each day.

Week 5: No takeaway food this week.

Week 6: Cook extra dinners to stock freezer.

Week 7: Read all labels during grocery shop.

Just as important as the goals are the rewards for achieving those goals. Make them non-food rewards. It could be things like a foot massage, a new book or CD, a bubble bath, a trip to the movies or for a family it might be a trip to the park or pool. If you achieve your goal for the week, then you get your reward. Keep it simple.

Step 2. Find the support you need

This is a huge part of managing any change in your life. Support is important to encourage you through the tougher times and to congratulate you on your successes. It is particularly important if you are looking to improve your whole family's diet as it will be a very tough road if you are the only one in the family committed to improving things. It needs to be a shared responsibility.

Let family and friends know what you are trying to achieve and ask for their help. Tell them why you are looking to improve your, your partner's or your whole family's diet. It may be weight loss, to boost your energy, to improve your sleep or just to feel better. It may be just the shared project you and your partner are looking for. If your family, friends or partner choose not to be supportive, then find a group who is. If you are looking to lose weight, there are many weight loss groups who meet regularly. If you are looking to improve your general health, look for a sporting or exercise group who shares your health aims. The importance of support and positive reinforcement cannot be underestimated when you are looking to make significant changes to your diet. Get out there and find some. It will make a world of difference.

Step 3. Look for comfort outside the pantry

Many people eat for emotional reasons rather than physical ones, so everything goes beautifully while the sun is shining but as soon as the storm clouds blow in, plans are abandoned. Emotion has ruined many good diets. Some people put on weight from their emotional eating. Others don't put on weight but their poor food choices could be doing just as much harm to their bodies – it's just not as obvious.

Make a list of some ways to comfort or distract yourself when you are tempted to stand at the freezer with a spoon in the ice-cream or open a small bag of crisps under the kitchen counter. You could put on a favourite song as loud as possible, go for a walk around the block or call a friend, anything that distracts you from making a poor food choice and undoing your good work. If you do want to have an ice-cream, chocolate or some other treat, by all means have one, but make it a conscious decision for the right reasons and part of your eating plan. That way it is one of life's pleasures and not something you will feel guilty about afterwards.

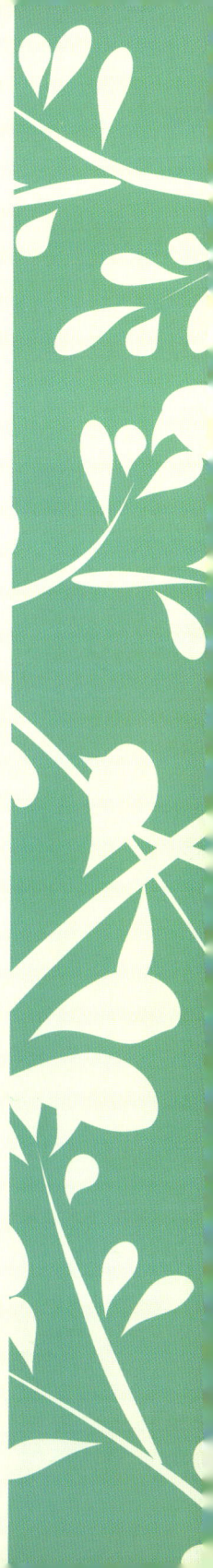

Step 4. Have a troubleshooting toolbox

Change is inevitable in life and even with all the best plans in place, something will happen that will throw things into chaos. This is where you can use your troubleshooting toolbox to get back on track.

Look at where the problem areas are for you or your family and find alternatives. It may be the after-school ravenous descent on the kitchen, the after-dinner kitchen phantoms looking for a little something extra or the moment you walk in from work and remember you haven't eaten since eight that morning.

Work out your eating Achilles heels and have a plan in mind. This may mean planning snacks better, making sure there is good food available when you or your family are hungriest, distracting yourself when you are prone to eating poorly, having stand-by dinners in the freezer if you have to work late, having five-minute healthy dinner options, having cold drinks ready for the children as soon as they walk in the door after school, whatever it takes to keep the good eating on track.

Step 5. Get your metabolism on your side

This is a very important step if weight loss is the aim of your diet makeover. Your metabolism is the rate at which you burn up food. There are a number of factors that could hinder or boost your metabolism and so affect your weight loss results. Genetics certainly plays a role. Everyone knows someone who lives on chocolate biscuits and cordial and never puts on a kilo! There are also other factors, some of which are outside your control. Your muscle mass, amount of activity, food choices, hydration levels, hormones, even your stress levels can affect your metabolism. There are some simple things you can do to help get your metabolism moving in the right direction.

Activity

Activity is the best way to boost your metabolic rate and burn calories faster. The more you move, the more efficient your engine becomes, the more calories you burn up and the more weight you lose. There is always an excuse not to exercise, so find something you love and stick to it. It is excellent for managing stress and also firing up your metabolism. Forty minutes, three to four times a week will really move things along.

Hydration

Recent studies indicate that hydration can increase cell metabolism, so drinking your two litres of water a day can actually have an effect on your ability to burn calories. If you are exercising, then your hydration needs will be even greater. Not drinking enough can also lead to confusing signals around thirst and hunger. We think we are hungry and eat something when, in actual fact, we just need a drink. Tally up how much water you have drunk before you reach for a snack and always have a bottle handy.

Thermogenic aids

Some foods are great for getting our metabolism firing. These are called thermogenic aids. They work slowly but keep things moving in the right direction. Chilli, ginger, garlic, onion and green tea are five top thermogenic foods. They all work to help fire the metabolism and manage cholesterol levels.

Blood sugar

Your blood sugar level is important for three compelling reasons: it affects how energetic you feel; how hungry you feel; and how you burn or store fat.

This is how it works: you eat a meal high in sugar or simple carbohydrates and your body releases a surge of insulin which is the hormone that deals with your blood sugar levels. The insulin tells your body that you have enough energy on hand and that it can stop burning fat and start to store it. It then works to move the sugar out of your blood to get levels back to normal. The surging insulin moves too much sugar out of the blood so your blood sugar levels drop below normal, you lose energy and look around for a sugar fix to give your blood an immediate top-up and reach for another chocolate bar. It's a vicious cycle. Keeping your sugar to a minimum and choosing complex carbohydrates over simple carbohydrates can stop this cycle and keep your metabolism roaring along.

Thyroid function

One function of the very busy thyroid gland is to regulate your metabolism.

It is highly unlikely that your thyroid is not working efficiently but if you have been a serial dieter in the past with poor results or have any symptoms of a poorly functioning thyroid gland, you may like to get your thyroid checked at the doctor to ensure it is working with you, not against you.

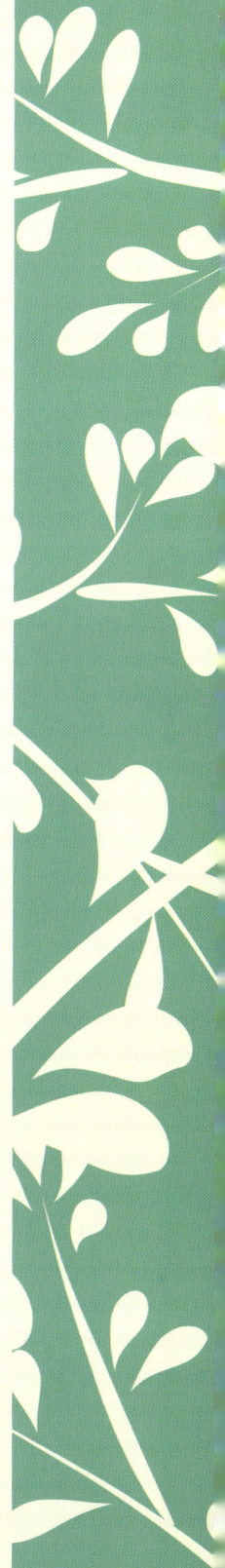

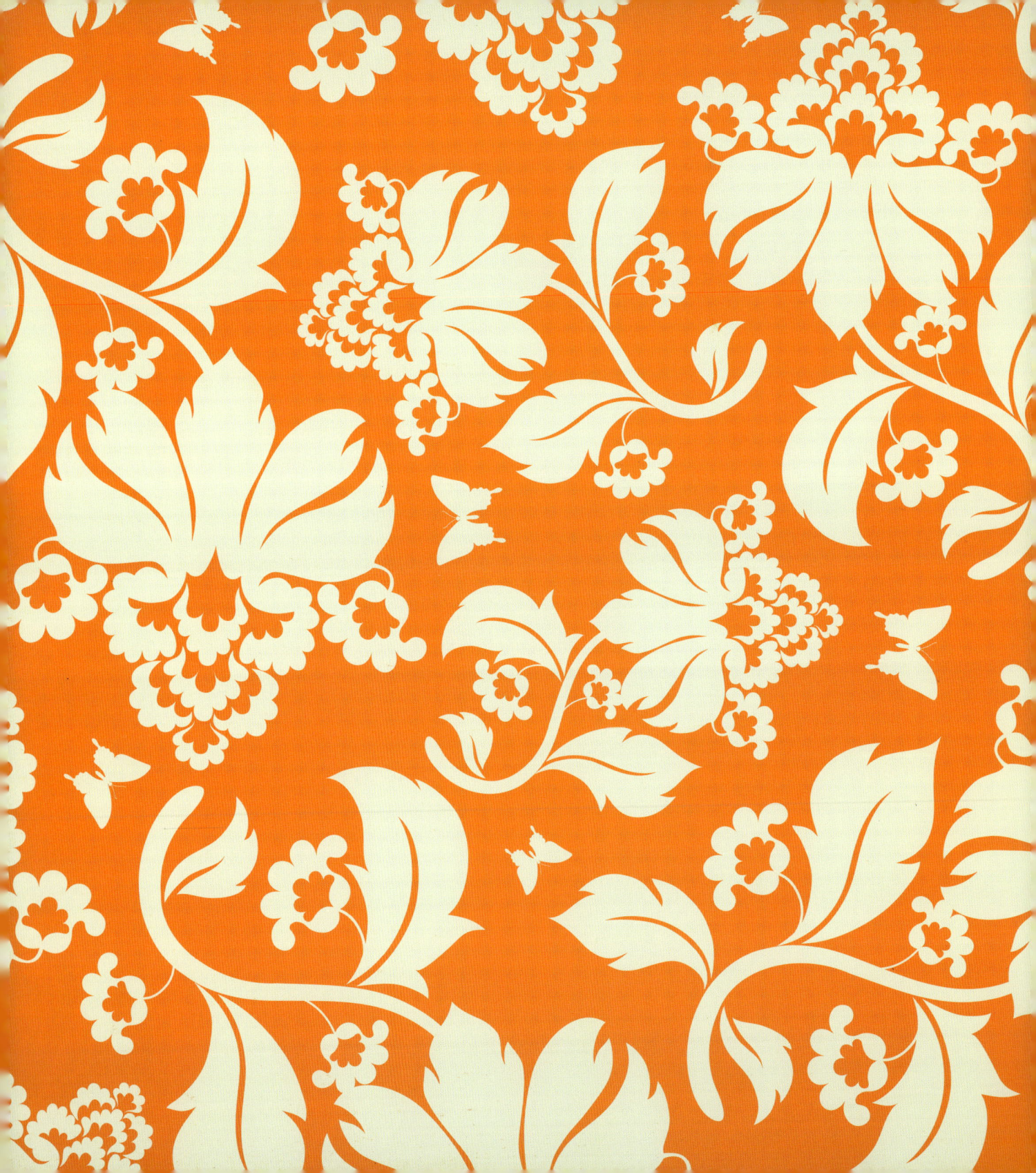

Breakfast

The weekend is when the fat breakfast comes into its own. We have time to prepare something a little special like streaky bacon, crispy fried eggs, thick slices of banana bread, creamy pancakes with lashings of syrup and cream; these are all weekend breakfast delights.

You don't need to give up your weekend breakfast feast, instead cook up the fab version. You won't taste the difference and you won't break the nutrition bank.

A Summer brunch for the girls

Have some girlfriends over and cook up a decadent brunch.

Eggs Benedict (page 56) with corn fritters (page 61)
  and wilted English spinach
Virgin bloody Marys (page 227)
Beautiful berry muffins (page 42)
Coffee and tea

A family Sunday brekky

Or make Sunday a family breakfast day, a time when you all sit together for an hour to eat and catch up on the week.

Creamy scrambled eggs (page 51)
Apple and cinnamon pancakes (page 46)
Rockmelon, banana and watermelon fruit platter
Banana smoothies (page 223)

Beautiful Berry Muffins

By using easy baking recipes, you can whip something up and have it in the oven within ten minutes. The other benefit of quick and easy recipes is that you can easily make just a small batch at a time and you don't have cakes hanging around the house that you are tempted to nibble on when you feel a little bored.

Serves: 6 • **Makes:** 6 muffins • **Difficulty:** easy • **Takes:** 10 minutes to prep, 20 minutes to cook

good quality vegetable oil
  cooking spray
½ cup (60g) self-raising flour
½ cup (75g) wholemeal self-
  raising flour
⅓ cup (80g) caster sugar
80g good quality spread, melted
1 egg, lightly beaten
150g frozen mixed berries (small
  berries only), defrosted and
  lightly mashed

Set the oven at 180°C. Lightly spray a six-hole muffin pan with the cooking spray.

Sift the flours together into a bowl, returning the husks to the bowl, and add the sugar. Combine.

In a small jug, combine the melted spread, egg and mashed berries. Add this mixture to the flours and stir until just combined.

Spoon the mixture into the muffin pan and bake on a shelf in the middle of the oven for 15–20 minutes. Test if cooked by inserting a metal skewer in the middle of one of the muffins. If it comes out clean, then the muffins are ready.

For a food nerd: Try these muffins with different fruits each time you make them. Tinned peaches, diced apple or even pumpkin would be great alternatives and help to boost the variety in your diet.

1 Serve: 6.3g total fat • 1.2g saturated fat • 748kJ (178 calories) • 27g carbohydrates • 3.6g protein • 1.8g fibre

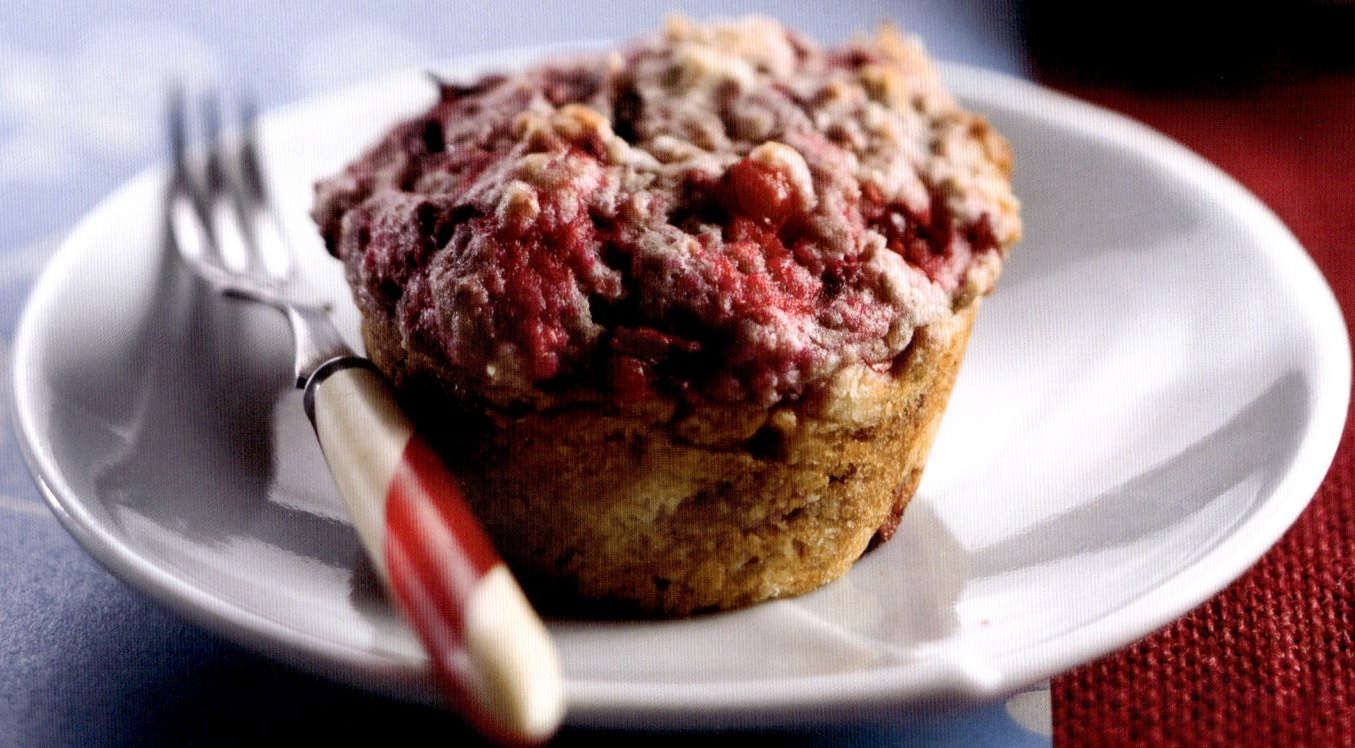

Orange Poppyseed Muffins

For some reason, the term muffin has a healthy connotation but most muffins are really super-sized cupcakes. To make these muffins fab, the fat has been cut down to only three tablespoons in total.

Serves: 15 • **Makes:** 15 muffins • **Difficulty:** easy • **Takes:** 20 minutes to prep, 20 minutes to cook

good quality vegetable oil cooking spray

1 tablespoon poppy seeds

⅔ cup (180ml) buttermilk or skim milk

1½ cups (185g) self-raising flour

1 cup (150g) wholemeal self-raising flour

¾ cup (165g) raw sugar

3 tablespoons good quality spread, melted

½ cup (125ml) fresh orange juice

1 egg, lightly beaten

2 teaspoons orange zest

Set the oven at 180°C. Lightly spray 3 six-hole muffin pans with cooking spray.

Soak the poppy seeds in the milk for 10 minutes.

Sift the flours together into a bowl, returning the husks to the bowl, and add the sugar. Combine.

In a small jug, combine the melted spread, milk, poppy seeds, orange juice, egg and zest. Add this mixture to the flours and stir until just combined.

Spoon the mixture into the muffin pans and bake on a shelf in the middle of the oven for 20 minutes. Test if cooked by inserting a metal skewer in the middle of one of the muffins. If it comes out clean, then the muffins are ready.

For a food nerd: Cut the sugar down to ½ cup (110g). This will make a drier muffin best eaten on the day is it baked, or you can freeze them for later use.

1 Serve: 2.1g total fat • 0.4g saturated fat • 571kJ (136 calories) • 26g carbohydrates • 3.2g protein • 1.1g fibre

Banana Bread

The bread in the name deceives us into thinking banana bread is a healthy café option. It is really just a heavy cake and, unfortunately, is often sliced very thickly making it a very large slice of cake for breakfast. Not a great start to the day. This banana bread is low in fat and sugar, is easy to make and freezes very well, so it can be pulled out and toasted for a quick, warm breakfast.

Serves: 12 • **Makes:** 1 loaf • **Difficulty:** easy • **Takes:** 10 minutes to prep, 45 minutes to cook

60g good quality spread
½ cup (110g) raw sugar
2 eggs, lightly beaten
3 very ripe bananas, mashed
1¾ cups (220g) plain flour
1½ teaspoons baking powder
½ teaspoon bicarbonate of soda

Set the oven at 180°C.

In a medium bowl, mix the spread and sugar together, beating until light and fluffy. Slowly add the eggs and mix well. Add the remaining ingredients and mix well.

Pour into a greased or baking-paper lined 23 x 11cm rectangular cake tin.

Bake for 45 minutes. Test if cooked by inserting a metal skewer in the centre of the bread. If the skewer comes out clean, then the bread is ready.

Serving suggestions: Serve with a Fruit smoothie (page 223) or some low-fat yoghurt.

For a food nerd: Use ¾ cup (110g) of wholemeal plain flour and only 1 cup (125g) of plain flour, add 2 tablespoons of wheat germ and serve it with small amount of nut butter.

1 **Serve:** 3.3g total fat • 0.7g saturated fat • 592kJ (141 calories) • 25.8g carbohydrates • 3.2g protein • 2.2g fibre

Apple and Cinnamon Pancakes

Traditional pancakes, filled with refined white flour, offer minimal fibre, are lacking in the energy giving B vitamins, contain no fruit and are bathed in butter while cooking… and that's before you add the toppings. They are just as yummy when made with wholemeal flour and cooked in cooking oil spray. Adding some fruit adds flavour, interest, texture and loads of vitamins, minerals and fibre. Berries, bananas or grated apple all work very well.

Buttermilk helps to make them extra fluffy, but if you don't have any, low-fat milk works very well too. For secrets to making the perfect pancake, check out the 'Cooking tips' on page 241.

Serves: 6 • **Makes:** 12 pancakes • **Difficulty:** easy • **Takes:** 5 minutes to prep, 20 minutes to stand, 15 minutes to cook

½ cup (60g) self-raising flour
½ cup (75g) wholemeal self-
   raising flour
1 teaspoon ground cinnamon
1 teaspoon sugar
1 teaspoon baking powder
1 egg, lightly beaten
1 small apple, grated
1½ cups (375ml) buttermilk
good quality vegetable oil
   cooking spray

Sift the flours, cinnamon, sugar and baking powder into a mixing bowl, and combine. Add the beaten egg, apple and half the buttermilk and combine. Add the rest of the buttermilk and stir well. Allow to stand for 20 minutes.

Lightly spray a frying pan with the cooking oil and place on medium heat. Spoon a tablespoon of batter into the pan.

Wait for bubbles to appear on top of the pancake, about 2–3 minutes, then turn over and cook the other side until brown. Remove from the pan and keep warm. Repeat with the remaining batter.

Serving suggestions: Serve with pure maple syrup, a teaspoon of low-fat ricotta and some sliced banana, berry compote (page 214) or one of the faux creams (use half of the amount in the recipe on page 214).

For a food nerd: Keep the apple skin on for extra fibre and add two tablespoons of wheat germ to boost nutrients.

1 Serve: 1.8g total fat • 0.7g saturated fat • 500kJ (119 calories) • 21g carbohydrates • 5.1g protein • 2g fibre

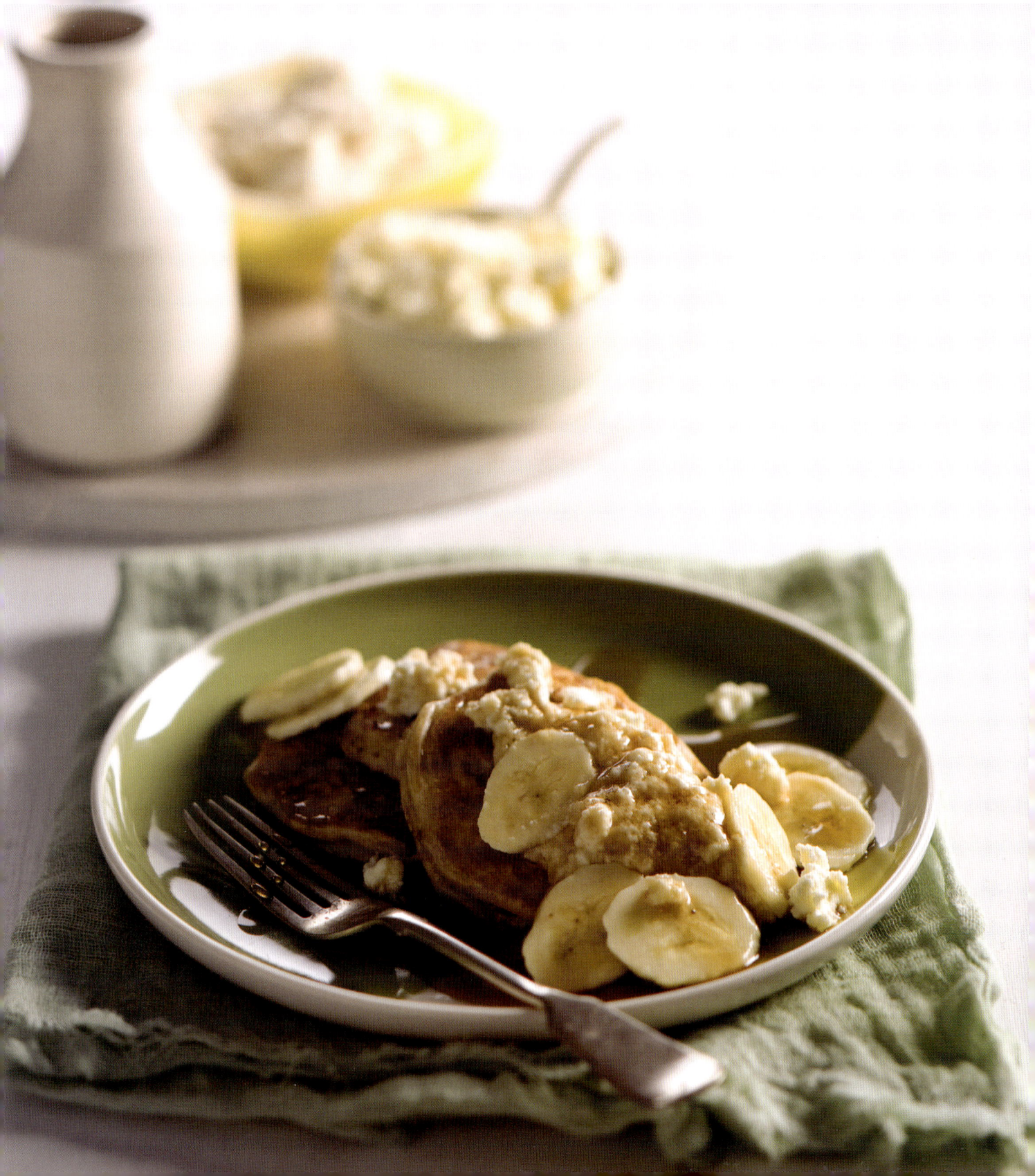

Ricotta Hotcakes

Low-fat ricotta and cooking with spray oil instead of shallow frying in butter makes these ricotta hotcakes a fab breakfast option. They are creamy and fluffy and look like the café version when drizzled with some pure maple syrup and low-fat vanilla yoghurt.

Serves: 6 • **Makes:** 12 hotcakes • **Difficulty:** medium • **Takes:** 5 minutes to prep, 20 minutes to cook

½ cup (60g) self-raising flour

1½ cups (225g) wholemeal self-raising flour

1 cup (250g) low-fat or extra light ricotta cheese

1½ cups (375ml) skim milk

2 egg whites

good quality vegetable oil cooking spray

Sift the flours into a medium mixing bowl. Add the ricotta and milk and combine well. Set aside.

In a large mixing bowl, beat the egg whites until they form stiff peaks. Gently fold in the ricotta flour mixture.

Lightly spray a frying pan with cooking oil and place on medium heat. Spoon tablespoons full of mixture into the pan. Wait for bubbles to appear on top of the hotcake, this indicates that it is browned on the underside. Turn over and cook the other side until lightly browned, then remove from the pan and keep warm. Repeat with the remaining mixture.

Serving suggestions: Serve drizzled with a small amount of pure maple syrup and topped with fresh fruit.

1 Serve: 0.8g total fat • 0.2g saturated fat • 731kJ (174 calories) • 30g carbohydrates • 12g protein • 2.5g fibre

Waffles

You need a waffle iron to make these but, like most small appliances, they are inexpensive to buy and make a very special breakfast treat. Eat them as soon as they are cooked so they are nice and crisp.

Serves: 9 • **Makes:** 9 waffles • **Difficulty:** medium • **Takes:** 10 minutes to prep, 15 to cook

1 cup (125g) self-raising flour
½ cup (75g) wholemeal self-raising flour
2 teaspoons cornflour
pinch of salt
2 teaspoons sugar
2 eggs, separated
375ml tin of low-fat evaporated milk
good quality vegetable oil cooking spray

Turn the waffle iron on.

Sift the flours and cornflour, returning the husks to the bowl.

Add the salt and sugar to the flours and combine. Set aside.

Beat one of the egg yolks until thick and pale, then add the milk and combine.

Add the egg-milk mixture to the flour mixture, stirring to form a smooth batter.

In a separate bowl, beat both the egg whites until stiff. Fold the egg whites into the batter.

Lightly spray the waffle iron with the cooking oil and spoon a small amount of the batter onto the iron. Cook until golden brown, about 4 minutes.

Serving suggestions: Serve with berry compote (page 214) and low-fat vanilla yoghurt, or with brightly coloured fresh fruit or sliced papaya and caramelised grilled pineapple with a dollop of low-fat Greek yoghurt.

For a food nerd: Add 2 tablespoons of LSA (ground linseeds, sunflower seeds and almonds) and wheat germ to the batter.

1 Serve: 2.9g total fat • 1g saturated fat • 580kJ (138 calories) • 22g carbohydrates • 7g protein • 1g fibre

French Toast

French toast is filled with whole eggs, full-fat milk and is cooked in butter. This version uses no milk, removes one yolk and cooks in olive oil cooking spray instead of the saturated-fat-laden butter. It is still crispy and delicious, and only takes five minutes, making it a great weekday breakfast. The protein in the eggs will keep you feeling fuller for longer.

Serves: 3 • **Difficulty:** easy • **Takes:** 5 minutes to prep, 5 minutes to cook

1 egg
1 egg white
3 slices wholemeal bread
olive oil cooking spray

In a bowl, whisk the egg and egg white together until smooth. Pour into a flat based bowl.
Soak each slice of bread in the egg mixture until saturated.
Spray a large frying pan with the cooking oil and heat to medium-hot. Add the bread slices and cook until golden brown on each side, about 3–4 minutes.
Serve immediately.

Serving suggestions: Serve this drizzled with 1 tablespoon of pure maple syrup, or sliced tomato and avocado, or red salsa. Add some fresh green salad leaves on the side, sliced seasonal fruit or a fruit smoothie.

For a food nerd: Use dark rye bread and add ½ cup of mashed silken tofu to blend in with the eggs before soaking the bread. For a bit of heat, add 3 drops of Tabasco and a dash of Worcestershire sauce to the egg mix. The chilli in the Tabasco helps to speed the metabolism.

1 Serve: 4.2g total fat • 0.9g saturated fat • 668kJ (159 calories) • 24g carbohydrates • 7.6g protein • 2.8g fibre

Creamy Scrambled Eggs

Creamy, fluffy scrambled eggs are lovely on a piece of warm toast. You can get the creamy richness by using buttermilk or light evaporated milk instead of cream and cooking the eggs in a small amount of a good quality low saturated fat spread rather than in butter.

Serves: 2 • **Difficulty:** easy • **Takes:** 5 minutes to prep, 5 minutes to cook

2 eggs

2 eggs whites

½ cup (125ml) buttermilk or low-fat evaporated milk

black pepper

1 teaspoon good quality spread

1 tablespoon chopped chives

In a bowl, whisk the eggs, egg whites, buttermilk and pepper together until well combined.

In a frying pan, melt the spread over low heat and pour in the egg mixture. Stir the eggs gently until they are just beginning to set. Remove from the heat immediately.

Sprinkle with fresh chives and serve hot.

Serving suggestions: Serve with steamed mushrooms, asparagus, tomato and English spinach.

For a food nerd: Add a few drops of Tabasco or some green chilli and 1 tablespoon of freshly chopped basil.

1 Serve: 6.6g total fat • 2g saturated fat • 520kJ (124 calories) • 4g carbohydrates • 13g protein • 0g fibre

Fibre friendly – easy ways to boost your fibre

Fibre helps to:
- Keep the digestive system healthy
- Lower blood cholesterol
- Assist with weight control
- Slow glucose absorption and maintain stable blood sugar levels
- Lower the risk of some diseases
- Keep your bowels regular.

Dietary fibre is found in cereals, fruits and vegetables. It is a type of carbohydrate made up of the indigestible parts or compounds of plants, which pass relatively unchanged through our stomach and intestines. Disorders that can arise from a low fibre diet include constipation, irritable bowel syndrome, diverticulitis, heart disease and some cancers. Don't fall into the trap of thinking that regular bowel movements exclude you from needing fibre in your diet – you still need it for all the other wonderful benefits it offers your body. When boosting your fibre intake, do it slowly, make sure you drink at least 2 litres of water a day and boost onions, shallots, leeks, oats, bananas and legumes in your diet as these are rich in oligosaccharides which work well with fibre to establish a healthy gut flora balance.

There are three types of fibre:

Soluble fibre – includes pectins, gums and mucilage, which are found mainly in plants, so in food we find it in fruits and vegetables. One of its major roles is to lower blood cholesterol levels. It also helps to reduce the risk of developing many serious diseases such as heart disease and bowel cancer and can help to reduce constipation. Soluble fibre forms a gel that slows down the emptying of the stomach and the transit time of food through the digestive system. Good sources of soluble fibre include fruits, vegetables, oat bran, barley, seed husks, flaxseed, psyllium, dried beans, lentils, peas, soy milk and soy products.

Insoluble fibre – includes cellulose, hemicellulose and lignins, which make up the structural parts of plant cell walls. A major role of insoluble fibre is to add bulk to bowel contents helping it to move through the colon and to prevent constipation and associated problems such as haemorrhoids. Good sources of insoluble fibre include wheat bran, corn bran, rice bran, the skins of fruits and vegetables, nuts, seeds, dried beans and wholegrain foods.

High fibre foods:
- Wholemeal and grain varieties of bread
- Wholemeal flour
- Jacket potatoes, new potatoes in their skins and baked potato skins
- Wholegrain breakfast cereals, eg wholegrain cereals, wheat biscuit cereals, bran flakes, unsweetened muesli and rolled oats
- Wholemeal pasta and brown rice
- Beans, lentils and peas
- Fresh and dried fruits – particularly if the skins are eaten
- Vegetables – particularly if the skins are eaten
- Nuts and seeds.

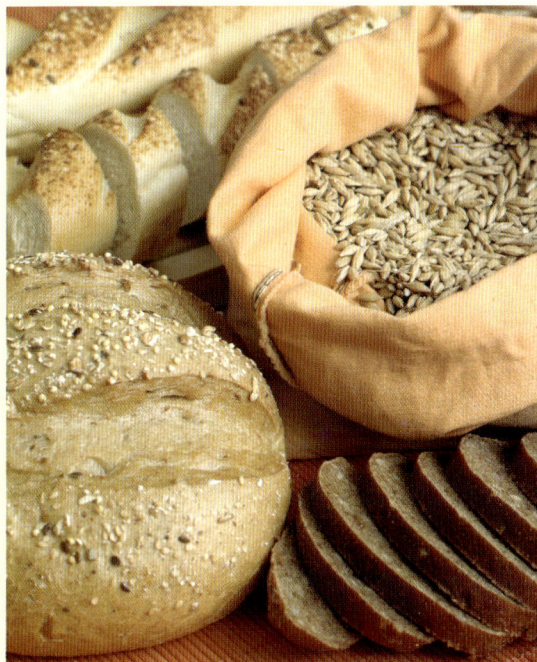

Resistant starch (RS) – is an exciting, new area of development in nutrition. Both the World Health Authority and the CSIRO recognise RS as a beneficial carbohydrate but the difference between RS and normal cabohydrates is that RS is indigestible and therefore passes through the digestive tract relatively unchanged and so is called a type of fibre. Like fibre, it promotes healthy bacterial growth in the gut and helps to keep blood sugars stable. It has less calories than other carbohydrates and is found in many foods including cold potatoes, rice and pasta. When these foods are cooled, their carbohydrate component changes and turns into RS, so for people looking to reduce their carbohydrates but unable to resist their potatoes and rice, a small serving of them cold can be a good option. For some sides rich in resistant starch, see the potato salad, harissa rice salad and pasta salad five-star sides recipes on pages 171 to 174.

Resistant starch foods:
- Legumes are the richest source. This means peas, lentils, navy beans, chickpeas, etc.
- Wholegrains
- Cooked cold rice, potatoes or pasta

We need around 30 grams of fibre each day, which in food terms could look like this: ½ cup of high bran cereal, ½ cup baked beans, 1 apple, 1 banana, ½ cup wholemeal pasta, 1 carrot and 1 cob of corn.

Most of us, however, eat around only 20 grams and so would benefit from a boost.

Easy Ways to Boost Your Fibre
- Use wholegrains. Replace white flour, pasta or rice in your recipes with the wholemeal equivalent or use half white half wholemeal. Add some whole oats to biscuits and slice recipes, and use whole oats for your porridge.
- Boost your legumes. Add some fresh parsley to a tin of four bean mix and serve as a salad, add a tin of cooked chickpeas, four bean mix, kidney beans or other legumes to any salad you are preparing, throw a cup of raw red lentils or chickpeas, butter beans or kidney beans into your soups, stews, casseroles and pasta sauce recipes.
- When you eat out, ask for wholemeal bread or rolls, have a fruit-based dessert and order a side salad or vegetables (with no added butter or salt).
- Boost your fruit and vegetable intake. Eat more salads or add an extra vegetable to your dinner plate. Fruit and vegetable juices contain very little fibre as it is removed in the juicing process, so opt for the whole fruit or vegetable.
- If you are eating rice or potatoes, cook them then chill them to allow the carbohydrate to turn into resistant starch.
- Use a fibre supplement. You could use a commercially prepared supplement or psyllium. These are not habit forming and do add to your total fibre intake, but they do not have the nutrients and other goodies that whole foods offer. So only use them short term or when you are away from home or don't have control over your food.

Spanish Omelette

Using the traditional method of making a Spanish omelette you would shallow fry the potatoes in a bath of oil and then add the eggs and more oil and shallow fry the omelette until set. It drips with oil and fat but is just as delicious when you cut the grease and make this lean version. It makes a great breakfast or a quick light lunch.

Serves: 2 • **Makes:** 2 omelettes • **Difficulty:** easy • **Takes:** 15 minutes to prep, 15 minutes to cook

2 small potatoes, unpeeled
4 eggs
2 egg whites
pinch of salt
¼ teaspoon white pepper
½ teaspoon dried oregano
olive oil cooking spray
1 small onion, finely diced
1 clove garlic, crushed
1 small tomato, diced
2 teaspoons flat-leaf parsley, finely chopped

Steam the potatoes until just tender. Allow them to cool before slicing them.

In a jug combine the eggs, egg whites, salt, pepper and oregano. Lightly whisk until combined. Set aside.

Make one omelette at a time. Lightly spray a small non-stick frying pan.

Over a medium heat, sauté half of the onion and garlic until soft. Spread the garlic and onion across the base of the pan and pour over half the egg mixture. Then arrange half of the potato slices over one half of the omelette and top with half of the diced tomato. Allow to cook until the egg just begins to set on top.

Fold the omelette in half and serve with the parsley sprinkled over the top.

Serving suggestions: Add a fresh fruit juice for breakfast or a rainbow salad for a light lunch.

For a food nerd: Replace the potatoes with a cup of steamed, diced pumpkin and sweet potato to boost the vitamin A and reduce the starchy carbohydrate content.

1 Serve: 9.3g total fat • 2.8g saturated fat • 1289kJ (307calories) • 37g carbohydrates • 21g protein • 5.1g fibre

Eggs Benedict

Eggs Benedict are a lovely decadent breakfast filled with fat and flavour. The fat is in the eggs yolks and the butter, so both have been cut in this recipe. The yolks are only in the sauce so only the whites are poached. This halves the number of yolks in the recipe but there is no noticeable difference in flavour. The butter is replaced by natural yoghurt which lends its creamy tartness to the Hollandaise sauce. The amount of spread used in this sauce is equivalent to how much you would spread onto your toast in the morning.

Hollandaise sauce has a reputation for being very difficult to make. I am no master chef and so was a little concerned when I hit the kitchen to test this recipe. I did it with no problems at all. If I can do it, you can too. It just takes some patience and confidence.

Serves: 4 • **Difficulty:** medium • **Takes:** 5 minutes to prep, 10 minutes to cook

4 eggs

40g good quality spread, melted

1 tablespoon white wine vinegar

1½ tablespoons low-fat or no-fat natural yoghurt

pinch of salt

pinch of white pepper

2 English muffins

4 slices leg ham, fat removed

1 tablespoon finely chopped chives

Separate the eggs, keeping each egg white in a separate glass or mug so that they can be poached individually later.

Place a glass or ceramic bowl over a small saucepan of simmering water. Don't allow the water to touch the bottom of the bowl as it is the gentle steam that will cook the sauce, not the actual water.

Drop the yolks into the bowl and whisk. Add 2–3 teaspoons of the spread and continue whisking until the sauce begins to thicken slightly. If the egg yolks begin to scramble, use a mitt to remove the bowl from the pan of water and continue to whisk until smooth and creamy.

Return the bowl to the pan of water. Add 2 teaspoons of the vinegar and whisk. Continue adding the spread and vinegar, alternating and whisking between each addition and allowing the sauce to thicken each time. Whenever the egg looks like it might scramble, remove the bowl from the heat to slightly cool, whisking all the time.

continued on page 58

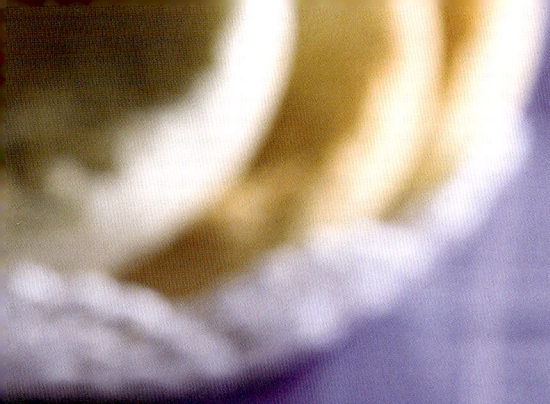

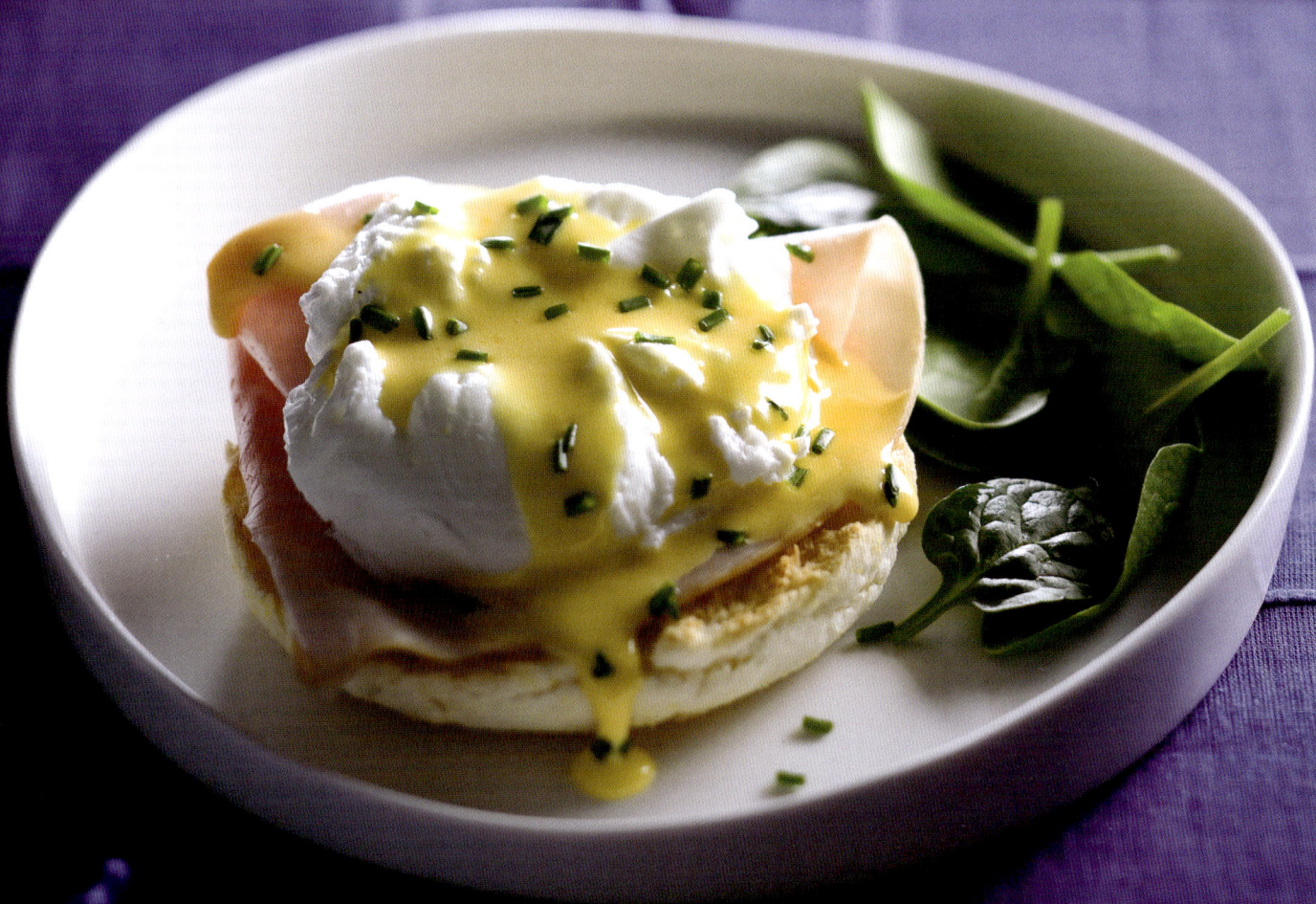

from page 56

When all of the spread and vinegar have been added, remove from the heat and slowly whisk in the yoghurt, salt and pepper.

Poach each egg white in the simmering water until just set.

While the whites are poaching, slice the muffins in half and toast. Lay one slice of ham on one half of the muffin, place a poached egg white on top and ladle over a couple of tablespoons of the Hollandaise sauce.

Serve sprinkled with the fresh chives.

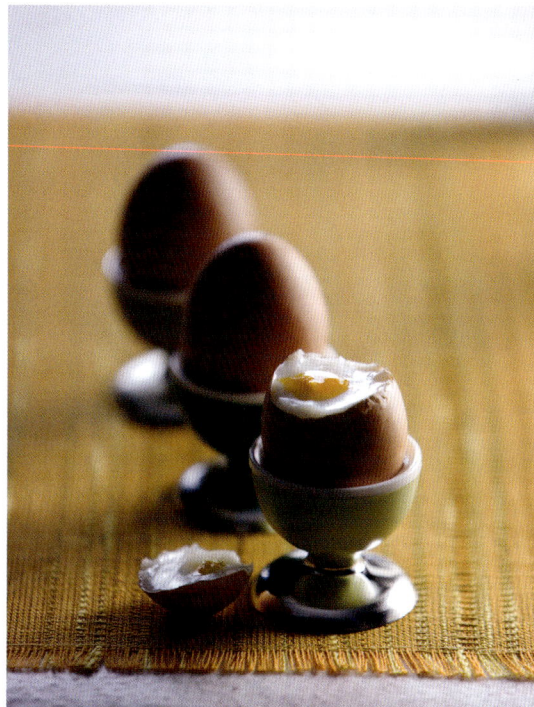

For a food nerd: Serve this with some fresh English spinach, raw or lightly steamed. If weight loss is not a goal, you could use whole eggs when poaching to get all of the goodness of the yolks.

1 Serve: 13g total fat • 3.3 saturated fat • 1025kJ (244 calories) • 14.6g carbohydrates • 14.7g protein • 0.8g fibre

Hash Browns

Most shop-bought hash browns are filled with 10–20 grams of cheap, nasty fat, lots of preservatives, and have already been fried once before being fried again. These madeover hash browns are crispy and tasty, and only take 20 minutes to make, from cupboard to plate.

Serves: 6 • **Makes:** 6 • **Difficulty:** easy • **Takes:** 10 minutes to prep, 10 minutes to cook

1½ cups peeled and grated potato

1 egg, lightly beaten

1 tablespoon extra virgin olive oil

Place the grated potato in a tea towel and squeeze out the moisture.

Put the potato and egg into a mixing bowl and combine.

Place the frying pan on medium heat and add the oil.

Spoon 2 tablespoons of the potato mixture into the pan, fashion it into a circle and allow to brown on the underside.

Once golden, about 3–4 minutes, gently flip over and cook the other side until golden.

Remove from the pan and drain on absorbent kitchen paper.

Serving suggestions: Serve with a poached egg, a slice of wholegrain toast and a glass of fresh juice.

For a food nerd: Use sweet potato for extra nutrients and less carbs.

1 Serve: 3.1g total fat • 0.6g saturated fat • 256kJ (61 calories) • 6.7g carbohydrates • 1.8g protein • 0.8g fibre

Kedgeree

Kedgeree is traditionally filled with cream. This recipe has no cream but still achieves the rich, creamy finish you look for in this dish. Try it with brown rice rather than white. You will not notice the difference but you will considerably increase the fibre and nutrients.

Serves: 4 • **Difficulty:** medium • **Takes:** 10 minutes to prep, 15 minutes to cook

1 cup (250ml) low-fat
   evaporated
   milk
¼ teaspoon pepper
¼ teaspoon turmeric
½ teaspoon cayenne
   pepper
pinch of salt
3 cups cooked brown
   rice
4 shallots, finely sliced
1 x 200g fresh salmon
   fillet, cooked and
   flaked
3 hard-boiled eggs,
   chopped

Slowly bring the evaporated milk to a boil. Add the pepper, turmeric, cayenne pepper and salt, and simmer for 4 minutes. Turn off the heat and allow the spices to steep in the milk for 10 minutes. Add the rice and heat through, then add half the shallots and salmon, and gently fold through.

Transfer kedgeree to a serving dish and top with the remaining shallots and chopped hard-boiled eggs.

Serving suggestions: Serve with some lightly steamed English spinach leaves.

1 Serve: 6.4g total fat • 1.7g saturated fat • 1302kJ (310 calories) • 44g carbohydrates • 18g protein • 2.6g fibre

Corn Fritters

Fritters are loaded with fat as they are deep-fried. These corn fritters are pan fried with cooking oil spray. Ensure you spray the pan lightly for each batch of fritters to give them a crispy finish. These are also great for brunch or lunch with some salsa on top and a small green salad on the side.

Serves: 8 • **Makes:** 16 fritters • **Difficulty:** easy • **Takes:** 10 minutes to prep, 15 minutes to cook

1 brown onion, finely diced
½ cup (60g) self-raising flour
½ cup (75g) wholemeal self-raising flour
½ teaspoon baking powder
3 eggs, beaten
2 egg whites, beaten
1 teaspoon paprika
1 tablespoon barbecue sauce
2 cooked corn cobs (260–270g), kernels sliced from cob
olive oil cooking spray

Mix together the onion, flours, baking powder, eggs, egg whites, paprika, barbecue sauce and corn until well combined. Allow to stand for 15–20 minutes.

Spray the cooking oil on the heated griddle pan.

Add 2 tablespoons of batter mixture per fritter to the pan until the pan is full of fritters. Cook until lightly browned on the underside, around 3–4 minutes, then flip and brown on the other side.

Serve immediately.

Serving suggestions: Serve with sweet chilli sauce or salsa, sliced avocado and a green salad.

For a food nerd: Serve with ratatouille (page 178) or rocket, pear and pea salad (page 158) to boost the vegetable content.

1 Serve: 2.1g total fat • 0.6g saturated fat • 424kJ (101 calories) • 16g carbohydrates • 5.5g protein • 1.5g fibre

Fry Up

The traditional fry up has 50 grams of fat, 14 grams of which are saturated! That is artery clogging stuff so consider where you can nip and tuck the fry up to make it leaner and cleaner without compromising taste. For example, have only a small amount of bacon and egg and instead fill up on the mushrooms, baked beans and tomatoes; buy low-salt and low-sugar baked beans and watch how you cook the eggs. Frying eggs in an oil bath will only end up on your tummy and hips. Use spray oil if you want to fry them, or poach or boil them if you are feeling very virtuous!

Serves: 4 • **Difficulty:** medium • **Takes:** 5 minutes to prep, 20 minutes to cook

4 tomatoes, at room
   temperature
½ teaspoon dried oregano
½ teaspoon dried thyme
pinch of sea salt
1 teaspoon balsamic vinegar
4 rashers 97% fat-free bacon
2 x 200g tins low-salt baked
   beans
olive oil cooking spray
4 large mushrooms, peeled and
   thickly sliced
1 teaspoon good quality
   spread
4 eggs
4 slices wholegrain bread

Cut the tomatoes in half and sprinkle each half with the oregano, thyme, sea salt and vinegar and grill for 6–7 minutes, or until warmed and slightly softened.

Place the bacon under a hot grill and grill to desired crispiness.

Gently heat the baked beans in a small saucepan, stirring occasionally.

Meanwhile, heat a frying pan sprayed with the olive oil over medium heat. Add the mushrooms and cook, stirring, until lightly browned, add the spread. Once cooked, remove the mushrooms from the pan (with any pan juices) and keep warm in a covered bowl.

Spray the frying pan with the olive oil.

Add the eggs to the frying pan and cook until they reach the desired consistency.

Toast the bread.

On each plate, place a slice of toast, baked beans, a rasher of bacon, an egg, mushrooms and two tomato halves.

For a food nerd: Add some English spinach, lightly steamed with a splash of white vinegar.

1 Serve: 16g total fat • 5.7g saturated fat • 2011kJ (479 calories) • 59.5g carbohydrates • 26g protein • 8.3g fibre

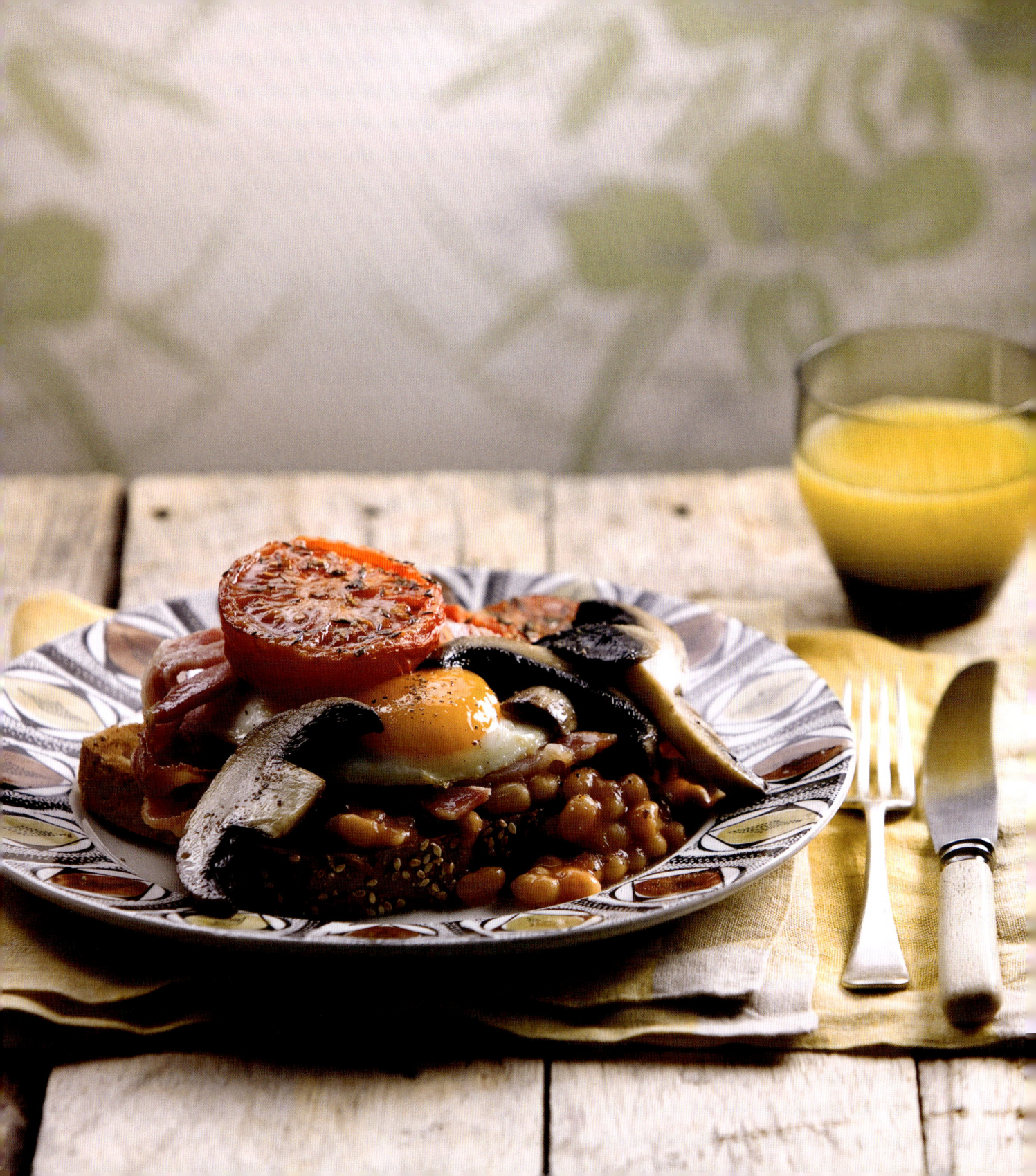

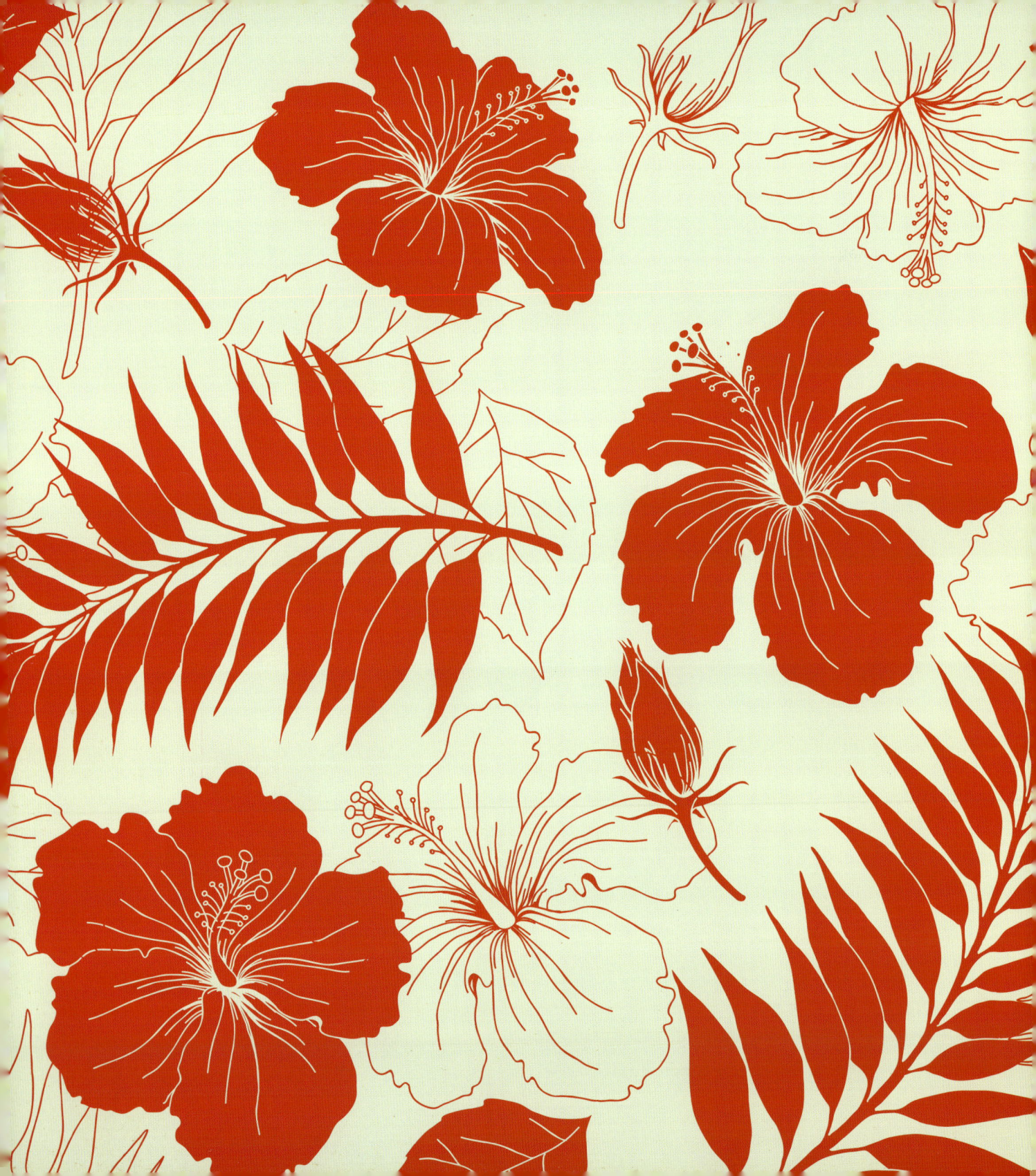

Lunch

What's for lunch? Perhaps some nachos, a pizza, a pie with some chips. It all sounds deliciously naughty but that's only because you don't know the fab secrets. Lunchtime is a wonderful time to entertain, particularly if you or your friends have children. Get some friends around to watch the footy or organise a celebratory birthday lunch.

Footy lunch for six

Birthday lunch for ten

Cream of Pumpkin Soup

Soups can sneakily hide lots of fat in their silky creaminess. Low-fat evaporated milk will give the soup the desired creaminess but is a whopping 95% lower in fat than cream, making it a fantastic choice.

Serves: 6 • **Difficulty:** easy • **Takes:** 10 minutes to prep, 35 minutes to cook

1 tablespoon extra virgin
  olive oil
1 tablespoon good quality
  spread
1 large onion, diced
2.5kg pumpkin, peeled and
  chopped
1 large leek, white part only,
  washed and finely sliced
3½ cups (875ml) low-salt
  vegetable stock
375ml tin low-fat evaporated
  milk

Heat the oil and spread in a large heavy-based stockpot over medium heat. Add the onion and lightly fry until soft. Add the pumpkin and leek and fry for 2 minutes. Add the stock and bring to the boil, then reduce to low and simmer for 30 minutes with the lid on, until the pumpkin softens and begins to break down. Stir occasionally.

Allow to cool slightly, then blend using a hand blender or blitz in batches in a food processor until smooth.

Return the soup to the pot, add the evaporated milk and stir well. Warm gently and serve.

For a food nerd: Add ½ cup (125g) of red lentils, a carrot and a sweet potato at the same time as the pumpkin to boost vitamin A, to give greater variety and to get closer to your daily 2&5.

1 Serve: 4.7 total fat • 1.3g saturated fat • 609kJ (145 calories) • 22g carbohydrates • 7g protein • 3g fibre

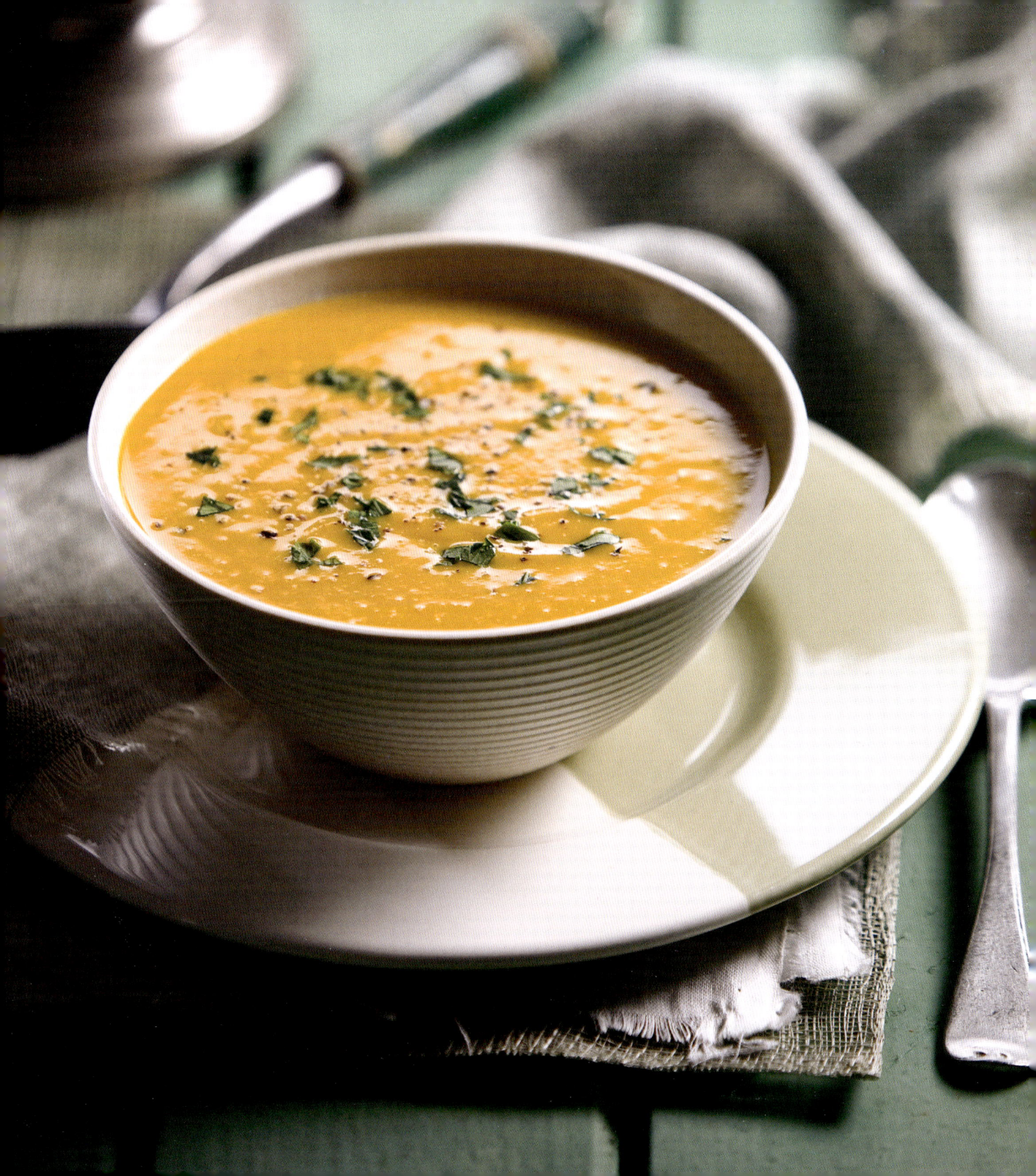

Cream of Leek and Potato Soup

This soup only just missed out on the fifth star because of its high carbohydrate content, but if you are not watching your weight, then it is a five-star lunch. The potato starch continues to thicken this creamy soup, so if eating it the next day you may need to add some stock to thin it before serving.

Serves: 6 • **Difficulty:** easy • **Takes:** 10 minutes to prep, 35 minutes to cook

2 medium leeks, white part only, washed

2 teaspoons extra virgin olive oil

3 large potatoes, peeled and roughly chopped

1.25 litres low-salt vegetable stock

375ml tin low-fat evaporated milk, warmed

2 tablespoons chopped chives

Finely slice the leeks, being careful to discard any dirt or grit.

Heat the oil in a large stockpot. Add the leek and fry for 2–3 minutes, or until the leek softens. Add the potato and stir well to coat in the leek and oil and cook, stirring constantly, for a further 2 minutes. Stir in the stock and bring to the boil, reduce to a simmer and add the evaporated milk. Cook gently, stirring occasionally, for 30–35 minutes, or until the potatoes are very soft and just beginning to fall apart.

Cool and puree the soup using a hand blender or blend in batches using a food processor.

Serve with the chives sprinkled on top.

For a food nerd: Use half potato and half sweet potato and add ½ cup (125g) of red lentils and an extra ½ cup (125ml) of stock to boost the nutrients.

1 Serve: 2.7g total fat • 0.9g saturated fat • 1789kJ (426 calories) • 43g carbohydrates • 9g protein • 4g fibre

Welsh Rarebit

Traditional Welsh rarebit is like a cheese fest, yet there is so much flavour in the Worcestershire sauce, pepper and mustard powder that using a stringy low-fat mozzarella and cutting the amount of cheese is not missed at all. This is a fast and delicious warming winter lunch.

Serves: 4 • **Difficulty:** easy • **Takes:** 10 minutes to prep, 5 minutes to cook

2 teaspoons extra virgin olive oil
1 teaspoon Worcestershire sauce
white pepper
1 teaspoon mustard powder
1 egg, lightly beaten
½ cup (50g) breadcrumbs
½ cup (75g) grated low-fat mozzarella
4 slices wholemeal bread

Heat the oil in a small saucepan over low heat, and add the Worcestershire sauce, pepper, mustard powder, egg, breadcrumbs and cheese. Stir the mixture until the cheese just melts. Remove from the heat.

Meanwhile, lightly toast the bread.

Spread the cheese mixture over each piece of toast and place under a hot grill for a couple of minutes, or until the cheese is golden and bubbling.

Serve immediately.

Serving suggestions: Serve with rocket, pear and pea salad (page 158) and freshly sliced tomato.

1 Serve: 6g total fat • 1.4g saturated fat • 655kJ (156 calories) • 17g carbohydrates • 5g protein • 2g fibre

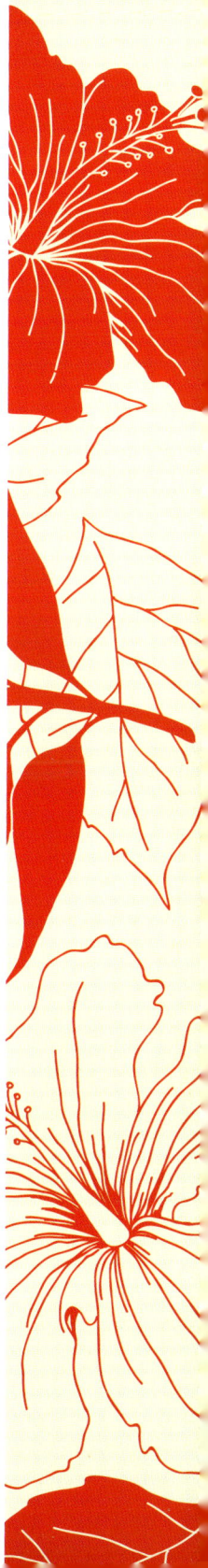

Caesar Salad

How can such a simple salad be so packed with fat? It is in the bacon, the croutons and the creamy dressing. You can bake the croutons, use fat-free bacon and only a small amount of flavoursome parmesan cheese to get the salad back on track, but it still needs the creamy dressing to be called a Caesar. The one below is creamy, but it's based on low-fat yoghurt.

Serves: 4 • **Difficulty:** easy • **Takes:** 10 minutes to prep

1 garlic clove, cut in half

3 slices one-day old
   wholemeal bread

olive oil cooking spray

4 rashers 97% fat-free
   bacon, all fat removed

1 large cos lettuce, washed

2 tablespoons finely
   grated parmesan cheese

Dressing

⅓ cup (80ml) low-fat or
   no-fat natural yoghurt

2 tablespoons lemon juice

1 tablespoon extra virgin
   olive oil

1 teaspoon Dijon mustard

1 garlic clove, crushed or
   finely chopped

1 teaspoon white wine
   vinegar

1 teaspoon
   Worcestershire sauce

Set the oven at 180°C.

To make the croutons, rub the cut side of the garlic clove onto the bread, then cut the bread into 1cm squares. Line a baking tray with baking paper and lightly spray with the cooking oil. Spread the croutons onto the tray. Place in the oven for 10–15 minutes, or until crunchy. Allow to cool.

Make the dressing by combining all the ingredients in a jug and whisking together well. Set aside.

Grill the bacon until crispy. Remove, drain on absorbent kitchen paper and allow to cool. Break into pieces.

Pull apart the lettuce leaves and tear into pieces. Place in a serving bowl and add the bacon, croutons and dressing. Toss to coat the salad in the dressing.

Serve topped with shaved parmesan.

For a complete meal: Add 100 grams skinless poached chicken breast torn into pieces, cherry tomatoes and rocket.

For a food nerd: Add a drained tin of 4 bean mix, delete bacon.

1 Serve: 9.5g total fat • 3.1g saturated fat • 852kJ (203 calories) • 20g carbohydrates • 11g protein • 4g fibre

Nachos

Nachos have so many problem areas, from the fatty fried corn chips to the sour cream and cheese on top. It is quite easy to do a makeover without losing the flavour, just go easy on the corn chips, use plain corn crackers or crispbreads, low-fat cheese, super skinny sour cream and fire up your metabolism with some jalapenos.

Serves: 4 • **Difficulty:** easy • **Takes:** 15 minutes to prep, 10 minutes to cook

12 thin, unflavoured rice or
  corn crispbreads
1½ cups (about 15 chips)
  low-salt, natural flavour
  corn chips
⅔ cup grated low-fat
  mozzarella

Sauce
1 brown onion, finely diced
2 teaspoons extra virgin
  olive oil
200g organic lean minced
  beef or chicken
½ teaspoon paprika
¼ teaspoon chilli powder
½ teaspoon dried mixed
  herbs
400g tinned tomatoes
1 tablespoon low-salt
  tomato puree
1 small red chilli, finely
  chopped
pinch of salt
pinch of sugar

Set the oven at 200°C.

First make the sauce. Fry the onion in a frying pan with the olive oil until translucent and soft. Add the beef or chicken and stir over medium heat until cooked through. Add the paprika, chilli powder, mixed herbs, tomatoes, tomato puree, red chilli, salt and sugar. Stir to combine well and bring to the boil. Reduce to a simmer. Cook, uncovered, stirring occasionally, for 10 minutes, or until the sauce thickens slightly and turns a deep red colour.

Meanwhile, arrange the rice or corn crispbreads and corn chips in four heatproof serving bowls and sprinkle with the cheese. Place the bowls on a baking tray and place in the oven for 2–3 minutes to melt the cheese. Remove from the oven and spoon the sauce over the warm crispbreads and chips, then top with one or more of the toppings. Serve immediately.

Serving suggestions: Serve with a rainbow salad (page 166) on the side. Toppings (all optional): diced or mashed avocado, red or green salsa (pages 164 and 165), finely sliced jalapeno or green chillies, finely diced spring onion or super skinny sour cream (page 88).

For a food nerd: Use low-fat natural yoghurt or cottage cheese instead of the sour cream, only corn thins, rice thins or rice cakes and no corn chips and be heavy handed with the chillies and fresh salsa.

1 Serve: 6.4g total fat • 1.7g saturated fat • 626kJ (149 calories) • 18g carbohydrates • 5g protein • 2.4g fibre

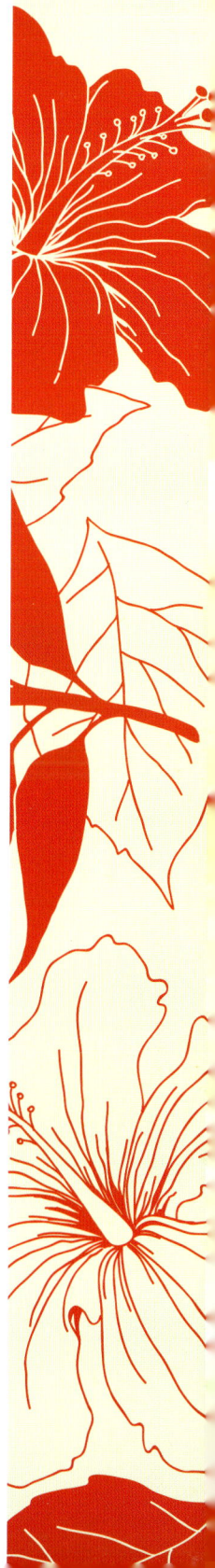

Club Sandwich

To make over club sandwiches, reduce the carbohydrates by using two slices of bread, not the traditional three, use lean chicken with the skin removed, fat-free bacon, boost up the amount of salad and dress it with a smart, low-fat mayonnaise that packs a flavour punch but is low in fat and kilojoules.

Serves: 4 • **Difficulty:** easy • **Takes:** 15 minutes to prep, 15 minutes to cook

4 rashers 97% fat-free bacon

4 eggs

8 slices wholemeal bread, toasted

2 tablespoons good quality low-fat mayonnaise

1 tablespoon barbecue sauce

8 lettuce leaves, washed and dried

2 large tomatoes, sliced

200g cooked chicken breast, thinly sliced

Grill the bacon until crisp.

Pan-fry the eggs in a non-stick frying pan until set. Remove from pan and set aside.

To build the sandwiches, begin by spreading a small amount of the mayonnaise and barbecue sauce on each slice of bread. Place a lettuce leaf and a couple of slices of tomato on each sandwich. Add a rasher of bacon, an egg and some of the chicken breast. Finish with the second slice of bread and cut diagonally in half to make two equal triangles.

Place a fancy toothpick in each triangle and serve immediately.

---

1 Serve: 14.9g total fat • 4.3g saturated fat • 1654kJ (394 calories) • 38g carbohydrates • 28g protein • 4.5g fibre

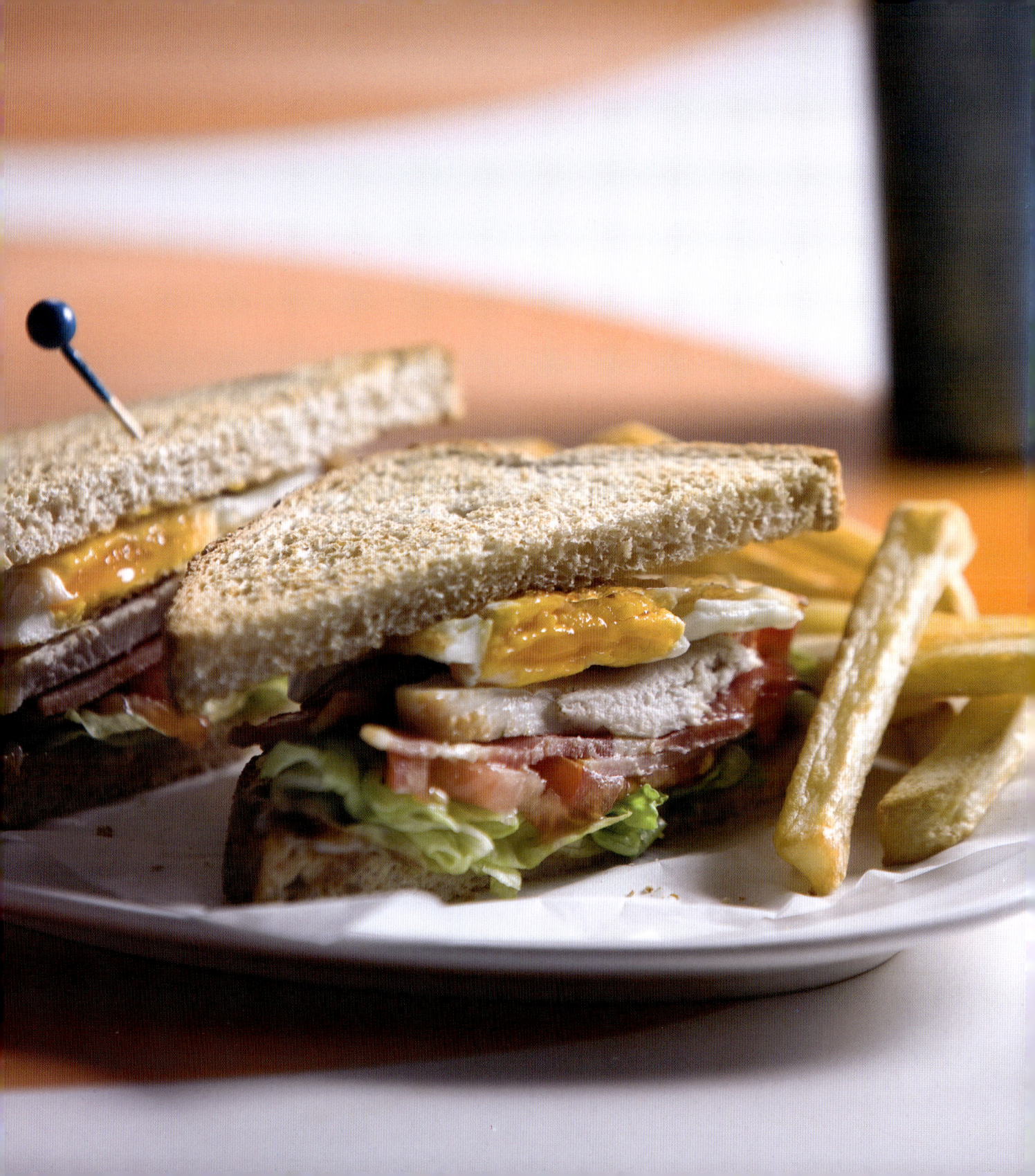

Hot Chips

For most of us, nothing beats hot chips. There is something about dipping them in sauce and the fluffiness of the warm potato inside that crunchy coating. They are just as yummy baked in the oven and they don't leave you with that greasy feeling afterwards (or that guilty one either).

Serves: 2 • **Difficulty:** easy • **Takes:** 5 minutes to prep, 30–35 minutes to cook

4 medium potatoes, peeled
2 teaspoons extra virgin olive oil

Set the oven at 220°C.

Chop the potatoes into 3cm length chips. Wrap them in a clean tea towel in a single layer to remove excess moisture.

Place the oil in a deep bowl and toss the sliced potatoes through the oil in batches.

Place the chips in a single layer on an oven tray lined with baking paper. Bake for 15–20 minutes, or until lightly browned and crispy, then turn them over and continue to bake for another 15–20 minutes.

Serving suggestions: Divide these two serves among four people and serve with a club sandwich.

1 Serve: 4.9g total fat • 0.7g saturated fat • 1546kJ (368 calories) • 74g carbohydrates • 8.6g protein • 9.4g fibre

Frittata

The ingredients in a frittata are not the only culprits in a fatty frittata. Shallow frying adds considerable fat and kilojoules. By using lots of vegetables and only a couple of teaspoons of olive oil (or spray cooking oil), you have a quick, nutritious, five-star meal that looks like something you ordered from a café.

Serves: 4 • **Difficulty:** easy • **Takes:** 10 minutes to prep, 10 minutes to cook

- 1 large (400g) sweet potato, peeled and diced
- 2 carrots, peeled and coarsely diced
- 2 teaspoons extra virgin olive oil
- ½ red onion, thinly sliced
- 1 garlic clove, minced or finely chopped
- 1 red capsicum, diced
- 6 eggs
- ½ cup (125ml) skim milk or low-fat evaporated milk
- 2 tablespoons finely chopped flat-leaf parsley
- 1 tablespoon finely chopped basil
- 1 teaspoon finely chopped thyme (or ½ teaspoon dried)
- 2 tablespoons finely grated parmesan cheese

Steam the sweet potato and carrot until just tender. Set aside.

Heat one teaspoon of the olive oil in a large heavy-based frying pan over medium heat and cook the onion, garlic and capsicum until softened. Remove from heat.

Whisk the eggs and milk in a large bowl. Add the sweet potato, carrot, parsley, basil and thyme.

Place the frying pan with the garlic and onion back onto low heat and spread the onion, garlic and capsicum evenly across the pan. Add the extra teaspoon of olive oil, then pour in the egg mixture and cook for 8–10 minutes or until just set.

If you do not have a heavy-based pan, the egg may not completely set in the middle and only be cooked on the bottom, in which case remove it from the heat, cover with a lid and set aside for 5 minutes. The residual heat will gently set the egg without further browning the bottom.

Sprinkle with the parmesan cheese and place under a hot grill until the cheese melts, 2–3 minutes.

Serving suggestions: Serve, warm or cool, with a green salad.

1 Serve: 10g total fat • 3g saturated fat • 1037kJ (247 calories) • 27g carbohydrates • 13g protein • 5g fibre

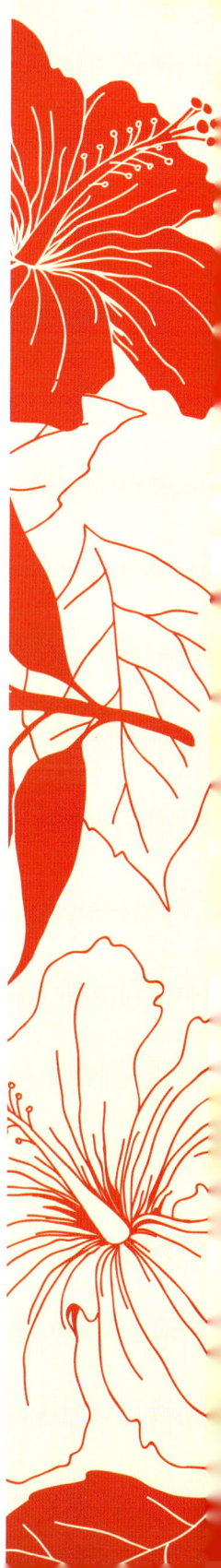

Cornish Pasties

Lard, the rendered fat of a pig, is where the crispy richness of a traditional Cornish pasty comes from and contributes to its 65 grams of fat (35 grams of saturated fat). By using reduced-fat pastry, brushing it well with beaten egg and cooking it in a hot oven, we still get the crispiness without all the saturated fat. Boosting the filling with vegetables and reducing the salt and fattiness of the meat makes pasties a good option.

Serves: 6 • **Makes:** 12 small pasties • **Difficulty:** medium • **Takes:** 15 minutes to prep, 35 minutes to cook

1 brown onion, finely diced
250g extra lean beef steak, fat trimmed, finely diced
pinch of salt
¼ teaspoon pepper
¼ cup diced potato
1 carrot, diced
¼ cup diced turnip, sweet potato or swede
½ teaspoon dried oregano
½ teaspoon dried thyme
1 tablespoon finely chopped flat-leaf parsley
3 sheets 25% reduced-fat puff pastry, thawed
1 egg, lightly beaten

Set the oven at 200°C.

Mix the onion, beef, salt, pepper, potato, carrot, turnip, sweet potato or swede, oregano, thyme and parsley in a bowl.

Cut each sheet of pastry into quarters. Round the corners off so that you are left with four circles from each pastry sheet.

Place a tablespoon of the mixture in the centre of each circle.

Brush the edges of each circle with some water and fold the pastry over the top of the mixture. Pinch the pastry edges together so that they are crimped.

Place the pasties on a baking tray lined with baking paper. Make a small slit to allow the steam to escape and brush the tops with the beaten egg.

Bake for 40 minutes, or until crispy and golden brown.

For a food nerd: For a vegetarian option, replace the meat with a tin of drained, mashed chickpeas.

1 Serve: 8.4g total fat • 3.7g saturated fat • 2612kJ (622 calories) • 21g carbohydrates • 16g protein • 1g fibre

Smart shopping and the 'latest nutrition breakthroughs'

With few exceptions, manufacturers are required to provide a nutritional breakdown of their food products. This is found on the nutrition panel at the side or the back of the packaging. The layout of the panel is standard across all products, but to fully understand the information given, you need to know some tricks of the trade.

All ingredients on a nutritional panel are listed in order by weight. The first three listed are usually the major three components of the food. Try to buy foods with a list of five or fewer ingredients.

Check where the food was manufactured or sourced. Our Food Standards Agency has made it mandatory to state the country of origin on the label. Some countries' food standards are far lower than ours and so the country of origin needs to be taken into account to ensure your food does not contain any hidden extras.

Sugar, salt, fat, fibre and added extras (such as thickeners and preservatives) are the five major things to look for on the label. See the translator below to make sense of the information of the nutrition panel.

One ingredient can have many different names. Sugar can be listed as sugar, sucrose, glucose, fructose, fructose syrup, maltose, corn syrup, honey, molasses, maple syrup, invert sugar, dextrose, golden syrup, lactose, malt, maltose. Fat can be listed as animal oil, fat, beef fat, copha, lard, milk solids, palm oil, shortening, tallow, vegetable oil, hydrogenated vegetable oils. Salt can be listed in the ingredients as sodium, baking soda, celery salt, garlic salt, MSG or monosodium glutamate (621), rock salt, sea salt or sodium bicarbonate.

Watch out for the nasty extras. Manufacturers use some ingredients to limit the growth of bacteria and other nasties, but some can be harmful. Avoid ingredients that have been hydrolysed or partially hydrolysed, E colourings ranging from E100–E180, the preservatives from E200–E285 and any product containing a long ingredient list filled with artificial ingredients, lots of chemical names, preservatives, flavour enhancers, emulsifiers, stabilisers, gelling agents or artificial sweeteners. The shorter and more natural sounding the ingredients list the better.

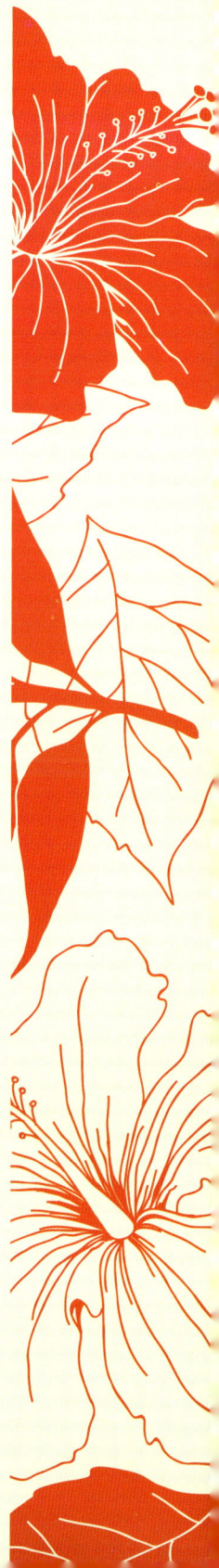

Sugar

Low in sugar: less than five grams per 100 grams.
High in sugar: more than 15 grams per 100 grams.

The sugar figure refers to the total amount of sugar in a food, including sugars from fruit, milk and added sugars. So, if you are choosing between two products with a similar amount of sugar but one product is filled with milk and fruit sugars and the other with added sugars, choose the milk- and fruit-rich product. You can tell if there is a lot of added sugar as it will appear high up on the ingredients list.

Fat

Low in total fat: less than 3 grams of fat per 100 grams (or 3% fat, 97% fat free) for solid foods.
Moderate total fat: 4–9 grams of fat per 100 grams.
High in total fat: 10 grams of fat per 100 grams. So if a food claims to be 90% fat free, that food is actually 10 per cent fat.

Low in saturated fat: 1.5 grams or less per 100 grams.
High in saturated fat: more than 5 grams per 100 grams.

On the panel, fat is often broken down to total fat, saturated fat and unsaturated fat (monounsaturated and polyunsaturated). A good product will have low saturated fat and no trans fats, as most of the fat will come from monounsaturated or polyunsaturated sources.

Salt

Very low in sodium: less than 40 milligrams per 100-gram serve.
Low in sodium: less than 120 milligrams per 100-gram serve.

Some labels only give a figure for sodium. You can calculate the salt content by multiplying the sodium content by 2.5. For example, 48mg sodium x 2.5 = 120mg salt. The daily maximum recommended intake for an adult is 6 grams. There are 3.2 grams in a ham sandwich, which shows you how easy it is to eat too much salt.

Claims such as 'lite' and 'low cholesterol'

Claims can be misleading. Look past the claims and consider what the food does contain rather than what is doesn't. Two common claims that can be misleading are lite and low cholesterol. Manufacturers must explain on the label exactly what their claim of lite and low cholesterol means. Lite can mean light in taste, colour, texture, or nutritional value; it does not always mean healthier.

Only foods derived from animals contain cholesterol, so 'no cholesterol' or 'low cholesterol' claims on foods derived from plants are meaningless

Translating the latest nutrition breakthroughs

News headlines often reveal new and exciting nutrition research breakthroughs which completely contradict what we heard the week before. Is fruit juice filled with sugar? Is avocado good or bad for you? Does a glass of red wine really promote better health? Sorting through this information is tough when all of the research seems to be conflicting. Who should we believe?

Headlines are written to be provocative and so arouse our interest. 'Eat a varied, balanced diet and you'll be fine' does not sell newspapers. They therefore often focus on cutting-edge research that is making huge claims from small studies or is yet to be corroborated by supporting studies. It takes a long time for research to completely prove or disprove a hypothesis. Keep this in mind when listening to the next round of breakthrough research and stick to a couple of simple rules as you filter this information.

1. Consider if the news is relevant to you and your needs.
2. If the news is relevant to you, take 10 minutes to jump on the internet and check the source and size of the study to see if it is credible or just a very early study looking into a new area.
3. Only make changes in your diet, if you hear nutrition news from a number of credible sources.
4. Remember that the principles of good nutrition always stay the same, eat a variety of foods and enjoy everything in moderation.

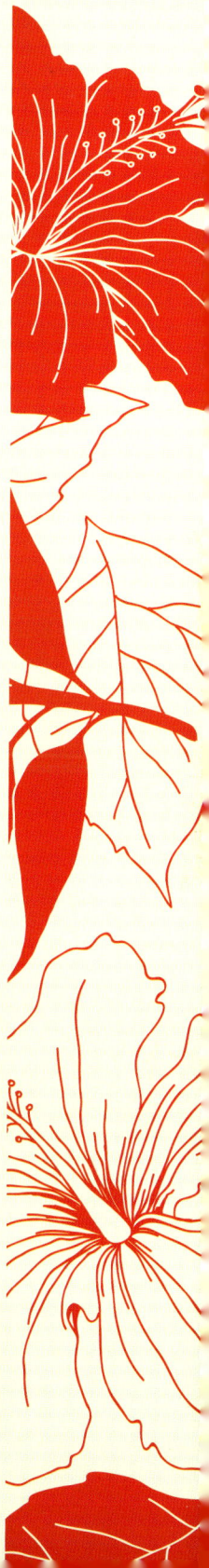

Quiche Lorraine

Bacon, eggs, cheese, pastry and milk give a traditional serve of Quiche Lorraine 56 grams of fat! That's four very fat reasons it needs a makeover. The recipe below uses low-fat bacon, filo pastry, low-fat evaporated milk and only a sprinkle of cheese, and yet it delivers the rich creamy flavour we look for in this dish.

Serves: 4 • **Difficulty:** easy • **Takes:** 10 minutes to prep, 20 minutes to cook

6 sheets filo pastry

olive oil cooking spray

4 rashers 97% fat-free bacon

3 spring onions, finely sliced

3 eggs

pinch of cayenne pepper

1 cup (250ml) low-fat evaporated milk

¼ cup (30g) coarsely grated low-fat cheddar cheese

Set the oven at 200°C.

Place one sheet of filo pastry in a 23cm round quiche dish and spray lightly with the cooking oil. Continue this layering procedure with remaining pastry, spraying each sheet lightly with the oil. Each time you add another pastry layer, rotate it slightly so that when all six layers are in the dish, the base and sides are completely covered with the filo pastry.

Grill the bacon until crisp, place on absorbent paper and dab slices to remove any remaining fat. Dice.

Mix together the bacon, spring onions, eggs, cayenne pepper, evaporated milk and cheese. Gently pour the mixture into the pastry case.

Bake in the oven for 10 minutes, then reduce the temperature to 180°C and bake for a further 20 minutes, or until just firm in the middle.

Serving suggestions: Serve with Moroccan bean salad (page 168) and a green salad.

For a food nerd: Use 100g of lightly steamed baby spinach and omit the bacon.

1 Serve: 8.2g total fat • 3.6g saturated fat • 756kJ (180 calories) • 14g carbohydrates • 14g protein • 0g fibre

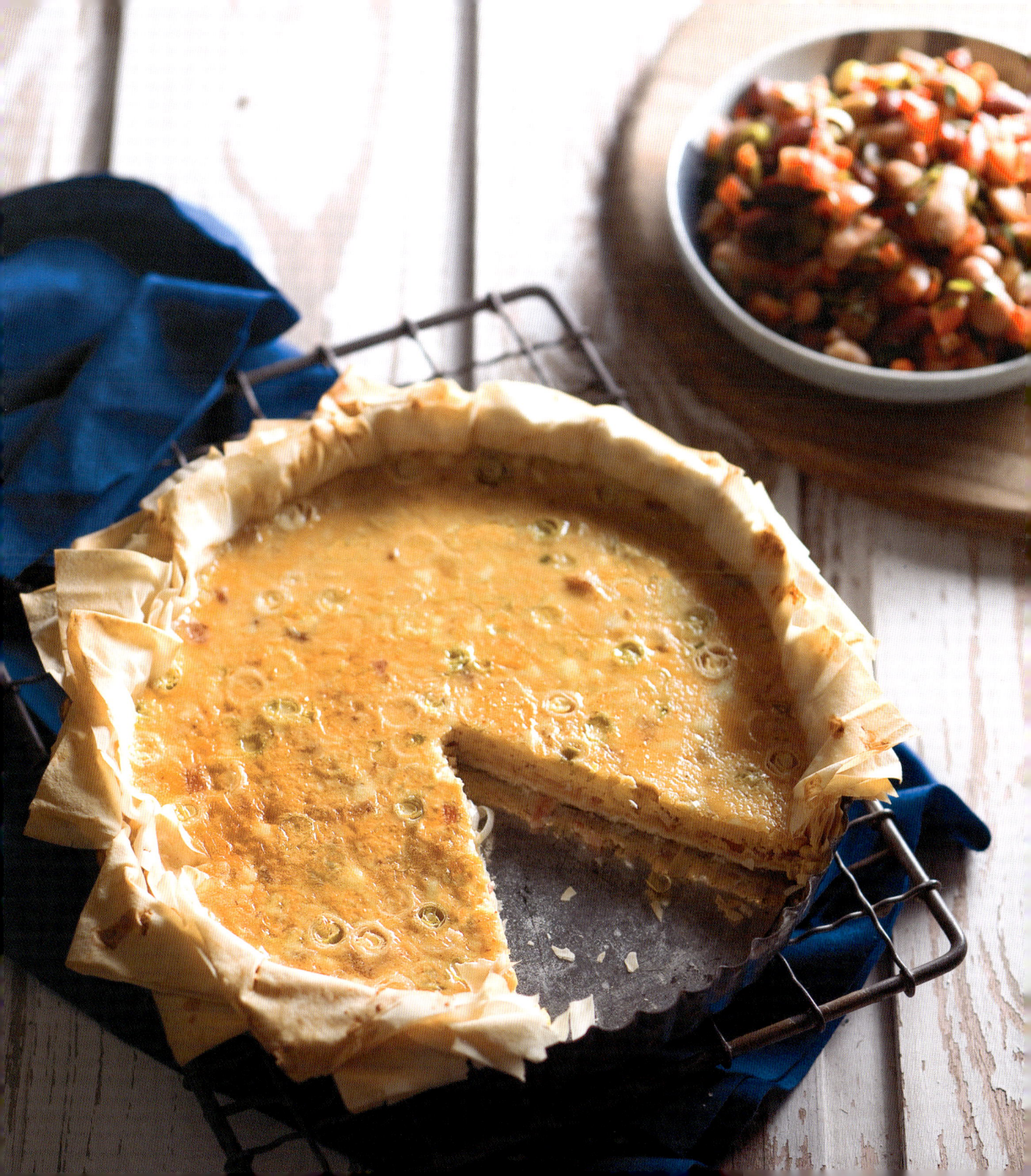

Sausage Rolls

From the flaky, butter pastry to the cheap, fatty sausage meat enclosed, the good old sausage roll is a super-bad fat choice. A traditional sausage roll has 33 grams of fat. By using good quality meat, adding grated vegetables, some herbs and spices and using reduced-fat pastry, they are transformed into a great choice. To make them an even better choice, you can make one large family-sized roll and so use a lot less pastry. You will need to bake the jumbo roll for longer until it is cooked through to the centre and then cut slices off to serve.

Serves: 12 • **Makes:** 12 large sausage rolls • **Difficulty:** easy • **Takes:** 15 minutes to prep, 40 minutes to cook

500g organic lean minced beef

1 small brown onion, finely chopped

½ cup (50g) breadcrumbs

2 tablespoons tomato sauce

½ teaspoon paprika

½ teaspoon dried oregano

½ teaspoon dried thyme

3 sheets 25% reduced-fat puff pastry, thawed

1 egg, beaten

Set the oven at 200°C.

To make the filling, combine the mince, onion, breadcrumbs, tomato sauce, paprika, oregano and thyme in a bowl. Set aside.

Cut one of the pastry sheets in half so that you end up with two rectangles. Place a line of the filling along one long side of a rectangle. Roll the pastry up so that you end up with a long shaped sausage. Repeat this process with the remaining pastry and filling until you end up with six long pastry sausages. Cut each long sausage into two smaller sausage rolls.

Place the sausage rolls on a baking tray lined with baking paper. Brush the tops with the beaten egg. Bake for 30–35 minutes, or until golden brown. Serve warm.

Serving suggestions: Serve with a large rainbow salad (page 166).

For a food nerd: Add wheat germ to the filling for increased fibre.

1 Serve: 13.4g total fat • 5.6g saturated fat • 1907kJ (454 calories) • 11g carbohydrates • 10g protein • 0.2g fibre

Hamburger with the Lot

Using good quality meat, wholemeal buns and loads of salad makes this a great meal for lunch or dinner on the weekend.

Serves: 4 • **Makes:** 4 hamburgers • **Difficulty:** easy • **Takes:** 10 minutes to prep + 30 minutes in fridge, 10 minutes to cook

250g organic lean minced beef

½ teaspoon Worcestershire sauce

½ teaspoon paprika

1 small brown onion, diced

1 egg, lightly beaten

1 tablespoon barbecue sauce

olive oil cooking spray

1 brown onion, finely sliced

4 egg whites

4 wholemeal hamburger buns

4 thin slices low-fat cheese

2 tablespoons barbecue sauce, extra

¾ cup shredded iceberg lettuce

2 tomatoes, sliced

8 slices tinned, drained beetroot

To make the burgers, place the beef, Worcestershire sauce, paprika, onion, egg and barbecue sauce in a bowl and, using your hands, combine well. Divide the mixture into four equal balls. Flatten the balls into a patty shape, place on a plate, cover with cling film and refrigerate for 30 minutes.

Spray a non-stick griddle pan with the cooking oil, heat over a medium heat and add the onion. Once the onion is softened, move to the side of the pan and add the burgers. Cook for 5–7 minutes, depending on thickness, until cooked through.

Move the burgers to the side of the pan with the onion and add the four egg whites. Cook until cooked through then place the eggs and the burgers on absorbent paper.

Meanwhile, slice the buns in half and pull out half of the bread part, leaving the roll crust with a small amount of bread inside. Toast.

On one half of each toasted bun, place a burger, then an egg, a slice of cheese, some onion and barbecue sauce. The heat of the onion and meat will melt the cheese. Add the lettuce, tomato and beetroot slices and place the other half of the bun on top.

Serve immediately.

For a food nerd: Omit the cheese and iceberg and add some grated carrot, radish, rocket and fresh red salsa (page 164).

1 Serve: 14.3g total fat • 4.9g saturated fat • 1596kJ (380 calories) • 40g carbohydrates • 24g protein • 4g fibre

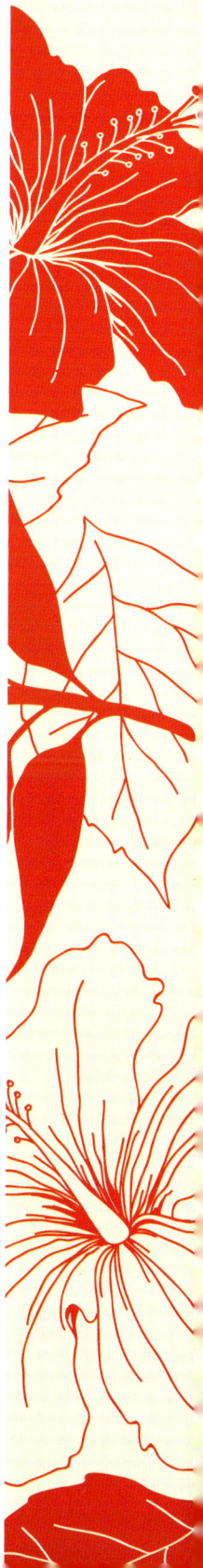

Pastizzi

It is the spread used to brush every single layer of pastry and the very cheesy fillings that put traditional pastizzi on the fat list. Using thin layers of filo pastry means that you don't need to brush them with any fat and low-fat soft cheeses, and herbs and spices in the filling make them creamy and tasty but keep them healthy and light. Pastizzi freeze really well and can be pulled out and popped into the oven for a warm lunch.

Serves: 4 • **Makes:** 12 pastizzi • **Difficulty:** medium **Takes:** 15 minutes to prep, 15 minutes to cook

1 large bunch English spinach, washed and roughly chopped
2 spring onions, finely chopped
2 teaspoons chopped mint
2 tablespoons chopped flat-leaf parsley
¼ teaspoon nutmeg
2 eggs
1 tablespoon tamari sauce
100g low-fat ricotta
100g low-fat cottage cheese
12 sheets filo pastry
2 teapoons good quality spread, melted

Set the oven at 200°C.

Steam the spinach until just wilted.

Place all the ingredients, except for the pastry and spread, in a bowl. Mix until well combined.

Fold one sheet of filo into thirds lengthways to make one long strip. Place a tablespoon of mixture at the bottom corner of the pastry strip. Take a corner of the pastry and fold it over diagonally to form a triangle. Continue folding to the end of the strip, so that you end up with a triangular package. Repeat the process until you use all of the pastry and filling.

Brush each triangle with the melted spread.

Place on a baking tray lined with baking paper and bake for 15 minutes, or until golden brown.

Serve immediately.

Serving suggestions: In summer, serve warm with a crisp salad and in winter, serve with a bowl of homemade vegetable soup.

1 Serve: 5.7g total fat • 2.3g saturated fat • 655kJ (156calories) • 14g carbohydrates • 13g protein • 0.6g fibre

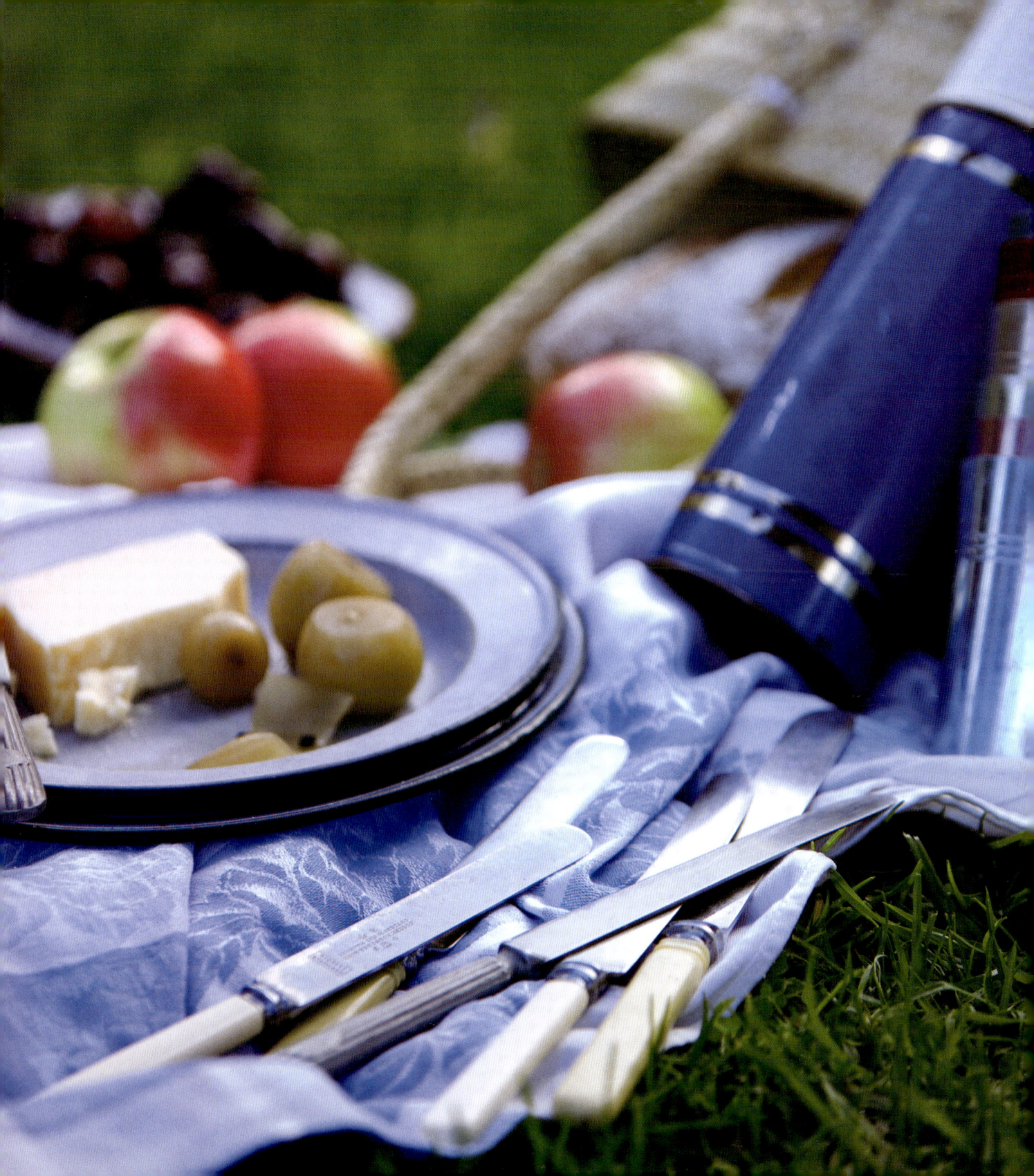

Pie and Sauce

You can't get more Australian than a pie and sauce. Using lean, good quality meat, a flavoursome reduced sauce instead of fatty gravy, and reduced-fat pastry halves its traditional 35 grams of fat. It is still quite high in fat so keep this for a special occasion. Grand final day would be perfect.

Serves: 5 • **Makes:** 5 pies • **Difficulty:** easy • **Takes:** 10 minutes to prep + 30 minutes in fridge, 10 minutes to cook

2 large potatoes, peeled and diced

2 teaspoons extra virgin olive oil

1 brown onion, finely diced

500g organic extra lean minced beef

1 tablespoon wholemeal plain flour

⅔ cup (160ml) vegetable stock

¼ cup (60ml) tomato sauce

2 tablespoons Worcestershire sauce

¼ teaspoon paprika

1 tablespoon chopped flat-leaf parsley

pinch of salt

¼ teaspoon black pepper

2 sheets 25% reduced-fat puff pastry

1 egg, lightly beaten

Set the oven at 200°C.

Steam the potato until soft.

Fry the onion with the oil in a non-stick frying pan until soft. Add the meat and stir until browned. Mix in the flour and cook for 1 minute, then add the stock, tomato sauce, Worcestershire sauce, potato and paprika. Stir and cook for 5 minutes, or until the sauce thickens. Add the parsley, salt and pepper and cook for a further minute. Allow to cool.

Roll out one sheet of the puff pastry to a thickness of 2–3mm and line four 10cm round pie tins.

Spoon the pie filling into the pastry-lined pie tins.

Using the remaining sheet of pastry, cut out four pastry pie lids, place on the filled pies and, with a fork, press the pastry edges together to enclose the filling.

Brush the pies with the beaten egg and place in the oven for 10 minutes. Reduce the temperature to 180°C and bake for a further 20–25 minutes until the pie lids are golden brown and crisp.

Serve with low-salt tomato sauce.

Serving suggestions: Serve the pies with a rainbow salad (page 166).

For a food nerd: Use mashed sweet potato instead of pastry on top of the pie.

1 Serve: 16.4g total fat • 6.4g saturated fat • 1491kJ (355 calories) • 45g carbohydrates • 15g protein • 4.3g fibre

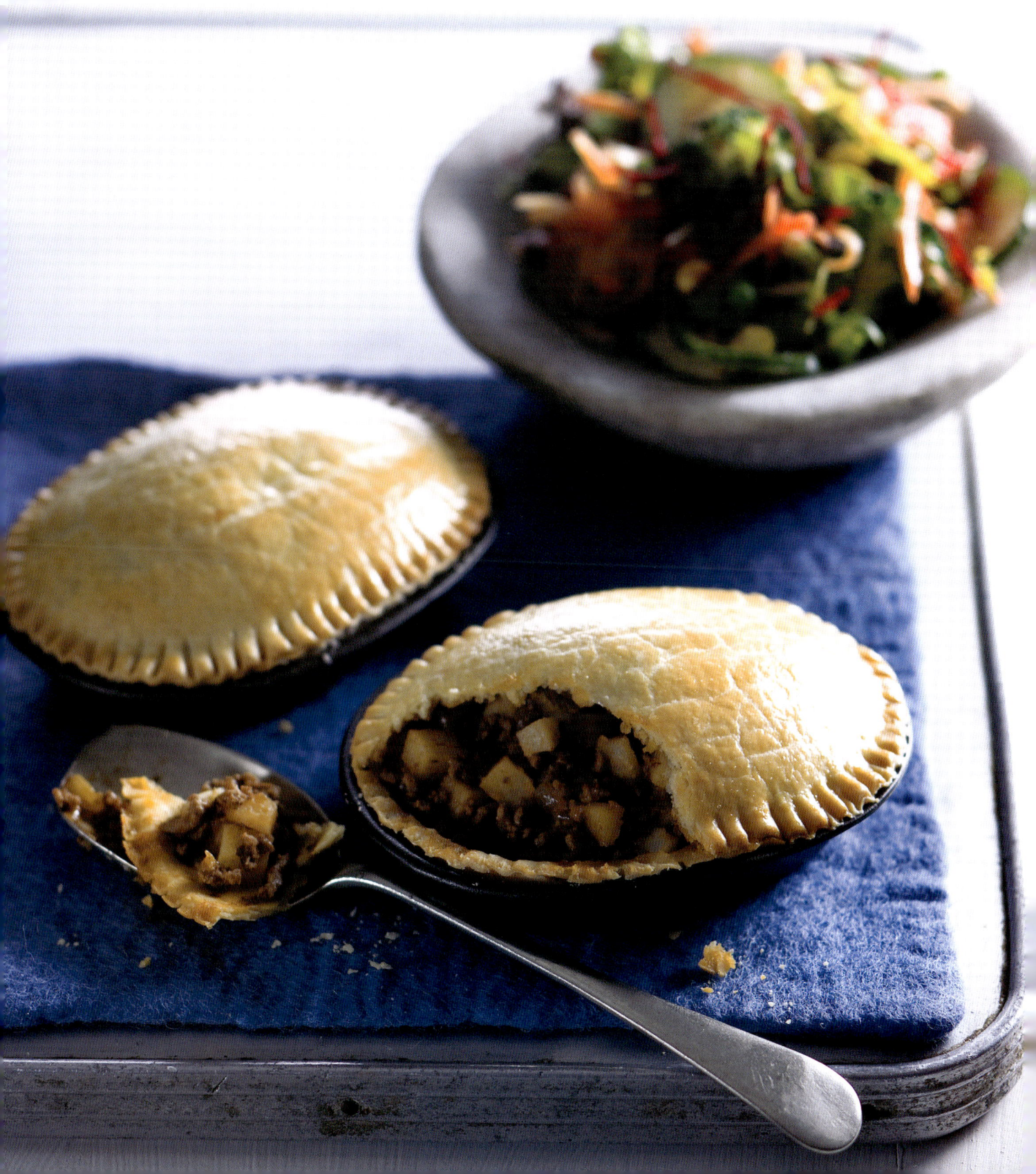

Wedges

Wedges are deep-fried and loaded with salt, then served with heart stopping amounts of fatty sour cream. It's easy to reduce the fat by baking them and serving them with a super skinny version of sour cream. It still gives you tasty wedges and some creamy dip but drastically cuts the saturated fat content.

Serves: 2 • **Difficulty:** easy • **Takes:** 5 minutes to prep, 30–35 minutes to cook

3 large scrubbed
   potatoes
olive oil cooking spray
¼ teaspoon spicy
   seasoning mix
Sweet chilli sauce to
   serve

Super skinny sour cream

2 tablespoons extra-light
   sour cream
2 tablespoons low-fat
   cottage cheese

Set the oven at 220°C.

Cut the potatoes into chunky wedges.

Line a baking tray with baking paper and spray with the cooking oil.

Place the wedges in a single layer on the tray and sprinkle over the spicy seasoning mix. Bake for 30–35 minutes, or until cooked through and lightly browned.

Meanwhile make the super skinny sour cream by mixing the sour cream and cottage cheese in a bowl until smooth.

Serve wedges with 1 tablespoon of sweet chilli sauce and 1 tablespoon skinny sour cream.

Serving suggestions: Serve with some lean grilled chicken and coleslaw (page 160).

For a food nerd: Mix the potato with sweet potato and parsnip to boost the colour and your vegetable variety. It is also a taste sensation.

1 Serve: 3.9g total fat • 0.6g saturated fat • 1915kJ (456 calories) • 96.7g carbohydrates • 11.2g protein • 12.2g fibre

Hawaiian Pizza

This Hawaiian pizza uses good quality lean ham and only a fraction of the usual amount of cheese. It has only a quarter of the amount of fat of the traditional version.

Serves: 1 • **Difficulty:** easy • **Takes:** 10 minutes to prep, 10–15 minutes to cook

1½ tablespoons red salsa (page 164) or shop bought

1 wholemeal Lebanese bread round

100g extra lean shaved leg ham

2 tablespoons crushed pineapple, well drained

2 teaspoons extra light cream cheese

¼ cup (35g) grated low-fat mozzarella cheese

Set the oven at 200°C.

Spread the salsa onto the bread. Arrange the ham and pineapple on top of the salsa and place small dollops of cream cheese around the pizza. Sprinkle over the grated mozzarella and place in the oven for 10–15 minutes, or until the cheese has melted and the base is crispy.

1 Serve: 9.6g total fat • 4.5g saturated fat • 1603kJ (391 calories) • 43g carbohydrates • 35g protein • 5g fibre

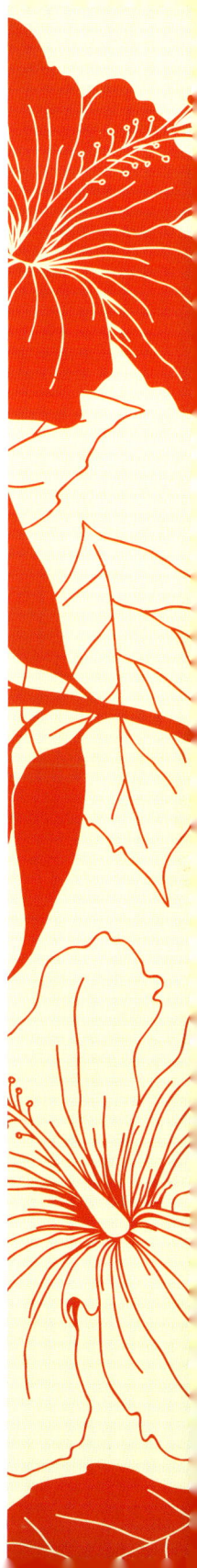

Vegetable Pizza

The cheesy toppings, fatty meats, oily grilled vegetables and the oil in the bases are the problem areas for pizzas. Reducing the cheese actually increases the flavour as you taste the rest of the toppings more than you do on a cheese-laden pizza. In this recipe, the cream cheese adds further richness and flavour.

Serves: 1 • **Difficulty:** easy • **Takes:** 15 minutes to prep, 10–15 minutes to cook

olive oil cooking spray

1 zucchini, thinly sliced lengthways

¼ small red onion, thinly sliced

8 thin slices eggplant

⅓ small red capsicum

1½ tablespoons red salsa (page 164) or shop bought

1 wholemeal Lebanese bread round

2 teaspoons extra light cream cheese

¼ cup (35g) grated low-fat mozzarella cheese

10 basil leaves

Set the oven at 200°C.

Heat a griddle pan and spray with the cooking oil. Chargrill the zucchini, onion, eggplant and capsicum on each side, then remove from the pan and set aside

Spread the salsa on the bread. Arrange the chargrilled vegetables on top of the salsa and place small dollops of the cream cheese around the pizza. Sprinkle over the grated mozzarella and place in the oven for 10–15 minutes, or until the cheese has melted and the base is crispy.

Roughly tear the basil leaves and scatter over the pizza just before serving.

Serving suggestions: To boost the protein, scatter ½ cup (90g) shredded poached chicken over the pizza. **For a food nerd:** Keep the meal vegetarian but boost the protein by serving with Moroccan bean salad (page 168).

1 Serve: 5.9g total fat • 2.4g saturated fat • 1516kJ (361 calories) • 67g carbohydrates • 17g protein • 16g fibre

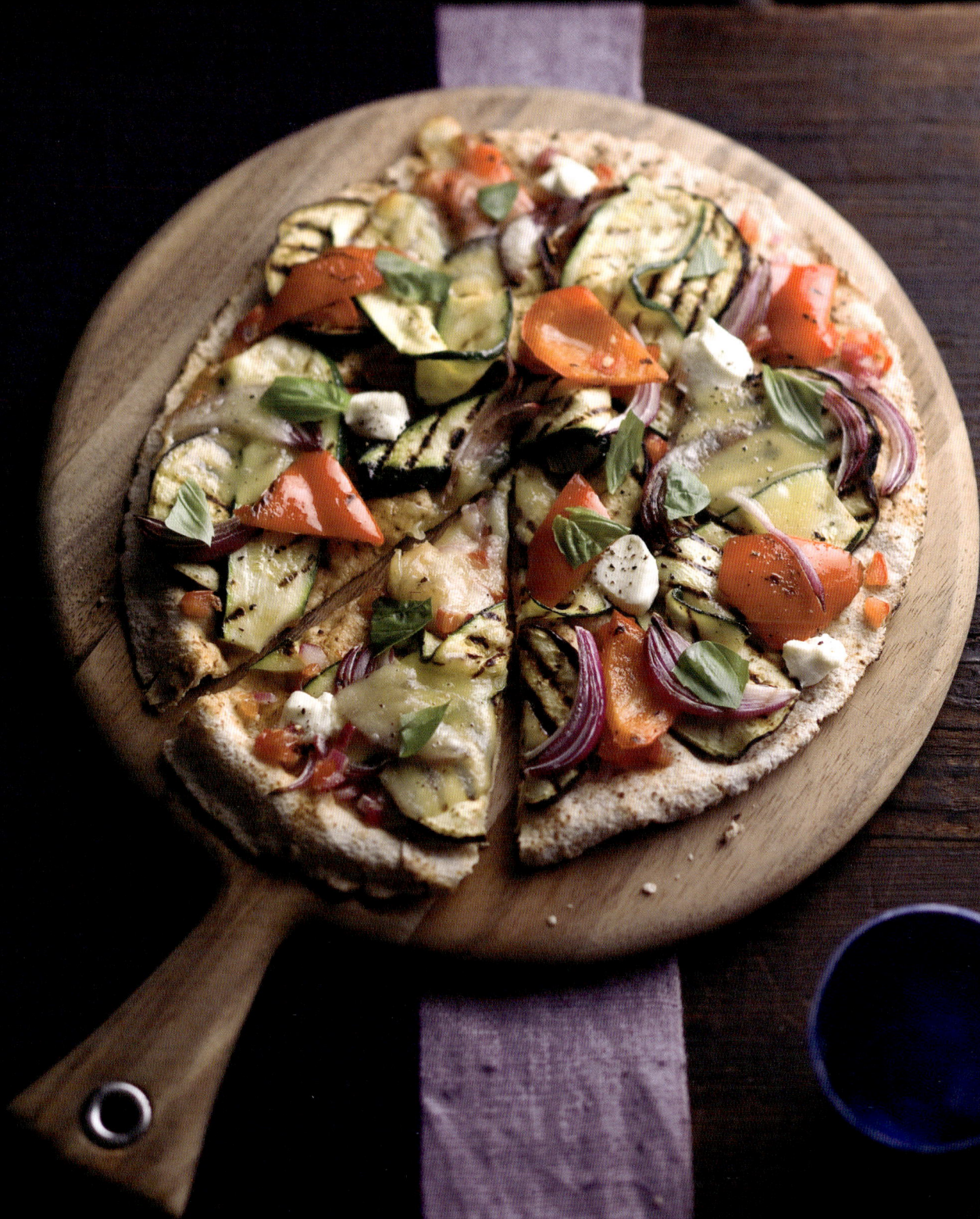

Fat lot of good: tricks for flavour not fat

Fat, sugar and salt are the cornerstones of flavour in most Western food, so when taking recipes from fat to fab, you are altering the balance and it can sometimes change or compromise the flavour. To boost the flavour, dig around in the flavour toolbox below. There is nothing tricky as all of the things are readily available at the supermarket, it's just a matter of knowing how to use them.

Flavour toolbox

There are two places where you can improve flavour in a recipe. First is in the method you adopt, for example, by cooking sauces for longer you allow the flavours to marry and the sauce to reduce, thereby naturally intensifying the taste. Also buy vegetables fresh and in season and only lightly cook them; there will often be no need for added flavours.

The second place to improve flavour is in the base ingredients, try these options:

INGREDIENTS	USE IN
Herbs and spices*	Italian cooking: flat-leaf parsley, oregano, basil, thyme, bay leaf. Indian cooking: curry, cardamom, turmeric, chilli, ginger. Thai cooking: Thai basil, Vietnamese mint, coriander, kaffir lime.
Aromatics (ginger, garlic, onion, shallot, leek, spring onion, chilli)	All cooking.
Sherry, wine	Sauces and desserts. Always boil to allow alcohol to evaporate.
Low-salt stock	Mashes and sauces to replace cream and other high-fat or high-salt ingredients.
Sauces**	Worcestershire: dressings, marinades, stews, rissoles and with grilled or barbecued meat. Hoisin and oyster: stir-fries, marinating meat and chicken. Tamari: replaces soy sauce. Fish: stocks, soups, salad dressings, dipping sauces and Asian dishes. Mirin: dressings, marinades and stir-fries.
Chutneys and relishes	Marinades, sandwiches, served with meat and chicken.

INGREDIENTS	USE IN
Vinegars	Rice wine: rice, Asian marinades. Balsamic: dressings, marinades, glazes and on sliced tomatoes, meat and fish. White: dressings.
Mustards**	Hot English: steak and very thinly spread on sandwiches, in mayonnaise and dressings. Dijon: sauces for fish or chicken, salad dressings. Wholegrain: lamb, chicken or salad dressings. American or yellow: hot dogs, potato salad, with eggs.
Tomato paste or puree (low-salt)	Soups, sauces, stews.
Dried mushrooms	Soups, noodles, stir-fries, risottos or rice for a smoky, rich flavour.
Horseradish	Egg dishes, salad dressings, with meat, in stock or with vegetables.
Wasabi	Sushi and other Japanese dishes.
Nuts and seeds (not peanuts)	Salads, stir-fries and in baking.
Anchovies	Sauces. Before using them, remove the bones and soak them in cold water for 30–40 minutes. Drain and pat dry before using. Just one-eighth of an anchovy dissolved in a sauce gives it a fantastic lively flavour.
Nut and seed oils	Replace butter and saturated fats.
Natural extracts and essences	Sweet dishes, drinks and baking.
Fruit zest	Marinades, for fish and chicken; in sauces, dressings and baking.
Rosewater and orange blossom water	Cakes, biscuits, sorbets, iceblocks, sweet doughs, most desserts, over oranges or fresh strawberries.

*   Woody herbs, such as thyme and rosemary, need to be added at the beginning of cooking to allow the flavours to be released. Grinding them in a mortar and pestle before adding can help to release flavours. Leafy herbs, such as parsley and basil, are best added at the end of the cooking process to preserve the delicate flavours. For specific herb uses, refer to the table on pages 240–241 in Resources. If you have an abundance of fresh sturdy herbs like thyme, curry and oregano, put them in a dark, dry place and dry them. If you have lots of leafy herbs like basil and parsley, blend them with a small amount of extra virgin olive oil and freeze them in ice cube trays, then transfer to snaplock bags for convenient year-round use.

** Use sparingly as most are quite high in salt.

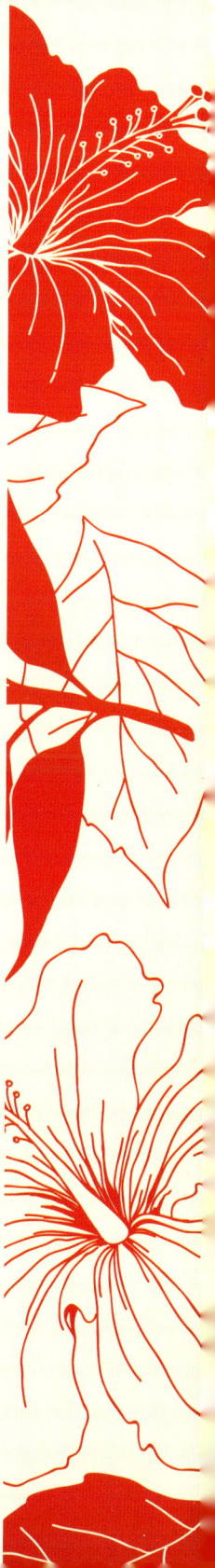

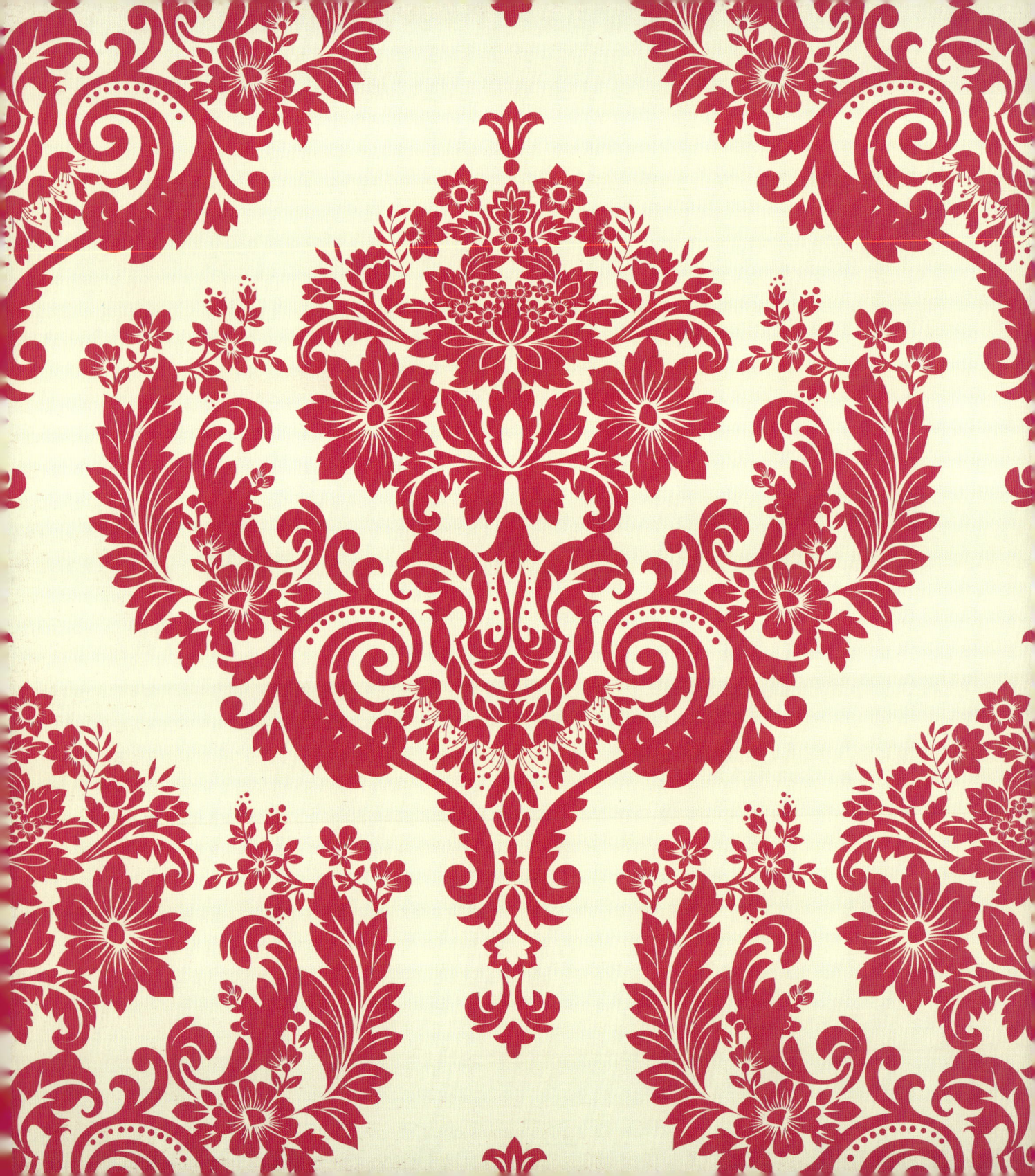

Afternoon Tea

There is something old fashioned and lovely about afternoon tea. We are so busy these days that by mid-afternoon we are lucky to get a cup of tea, let alone sit down and enjoy some delicious refreshments. That makes afternoon tea even more special when you do take the time.

Why not hold a high tea for the girls or a spring garden party for family and friends?

High tea for the girls

Cucumber sandwiches

Mini quiche Lorraines (page 80)

High tea scones (page 96)

Lisa's butterfly cakes (page 98)

Truffles (page 102)

Platter of raspberries, blueberries and strawberries

Fresh mint tea

Spring garden tea for family and friends

Lemon tarts (page 104)

Chocolate banana cupcakes (page 105)

Apple tea cake (page 108)

Vanilla slice (page 110)

Cherry, pineapple, honeydew melon platter

Lemon spritzers (page 231)

High Tea Scones

Scones recipes vary greatly. Most of them contain butter, cream and full-cream milk. This lean version below has none of these. The fluffiness comes from the spread and how the dough is handled. The secret to great scones is keeping the dough cold. Use cold low-fat spread, stir the dough with a cold butter knife and handle it as little as possible. The weather also has an effect on your dough. Some days you may need to add a touch more milk to help your dough come together. Always add liquid slowly to ensure just the right amount is added.

Makes: 15 scones • **Difficulty:** easy • **Takes:** 15 minutes to prep, 15 minutes to cook

2 cups (250g) self-raising flour
1½ tablespoons good quality spread
⅔ cup (160ml) buttermilk
1 egg white, lightly beaten

Set the oven at 200°C.

Sift the flour twice into a bowl.

Using your fingertips, rub the spread into the flour until it resembles breadcrumbs. Gradually add the buttermilk, while mixing with a cold butter knife until it is a soft dough. Place the dough on a lightly floured surface and knead until just smooth.

Roll out to 3cm thickness and cut out scones with a scone cutter or use a knife to cut into square scones.

Place the scones very close together on a a baking-paper lined or lightly floured 20cm square baking tin. Brush the tops of the scones with the egg white.

Bake for 10–15 minutes, or until lightly browned on top.

For a food nerd: Add 2 tablespoons of wheat germ, replace 1 of the cups of white flour with wholemeal flour and add ⅔ cup of dried fruit such as apricots, chopped dates or sultanas.

1 Serve: 1g total fat • 0.2g saturated fat • 298kJ (71 calories) • 13g carbohydrates • 2g protein • 0.5g fibre

Brownies

With 14 grams of fat a piece, brownies are one of the ultimate indulgence foods. They are filled with nuts, chocolate and butter. This version gets the chocolate flavour from cocoa and only uses 100 grams of reduced-fat spread.

Makes: 24 brownies • **Difficulty:** easy • **Takes:** 10 minutes to prep, 20 minutes to cook

1 cup (125g) plain flour

1 cup (150g) wholemeal plain flour

2 tablespoons unsweetened cocoa powder

½ cup (110g) raw sugar

¼ cup (30g) walnut pieces, roughly chopped

1 egg, lightly beaten

100g good quality reduced-fat spread, melted

1 teaspoon natural vanilla extract

2 teaspoons icing sugar, to dust

Set the oven at 180°C.

Sift the flours and cocoa into a bowl. Add the sugar and walnut pieces and stir well.

In a small jug, combine the egg, melted spread and vanilla. Add to the dry ingredients and mix well.

Spoon the mixture into a baking-paper lined 20cm square cake tin. Bake in the oven for 20–25 minutes until lightly browned and firm.

Remove from the oven and allow to cool in the tin. Turn out and dust with the sifted icing sugar. Cut into 24 bars.

For a food nerd: If you are not watching your weight, replace 1 cup of the flour with almond meal. It will increase the overall fat content of the brownies, but will boost the nutrition, especially the protein and calcium.

1 Serve: 2.8g total fat • 0.5g saturated fat • 328kJ (78 calories) • 12g carbohydrates • 2g protein • 0.3g fibre

Lisa's Butterfly Cakes

These cakes are based on a sponge recipe, which is why they are light and fluffy but have next to no fat. This recipe uses caster sugar, as texture is so important in a butterfly cake, but you could use raw sugar. You will see that the recipe is high in sugar. With no added fat in this cake mixture, there is no way to reduce the sugar any further. Because they are so low in fat, they are best eaten on the day they are made as they will begin to dry out the next day.

Makes: 12 little cakes • **Difficulty:** medium • **Takes:** 15 minutes to prep, 15 minutes to cook

1 cup (125g) self-raising flour
2 eggs
⅔ cup (145g) caster sugar
3 tablespoons skim milk
1 teaspoons natural vanilla
 extract
good quality vegetable oil
 cooking spray

Topping
3½ tablespoons strawberry jam
1 quantity ricotta cream (page
 217) or faux cream (page 217)
icing sugar, to dust

Set the oven at 180°C and place a 12-hole muffin pan on the middle shelf.

Sift the flour into a bowl twice and set aside.

Place the eggs and sugar in a bowl and beat well until thick and pale. Add the flour, milk and vanilla. Stir until well combined.

Using an oven mitt, remove the hot muffin pan from the oven and spray with cooking oil. Carefully spoon the mixture into the sprayed hot muffin pan (do not use paper cupcake cases), filling each hole about two-thirds. Place in the oven and cook for 8 minutes or until just cooked through. Test if cooked by inserting a metal skewer in the middle of one of the cakes. If it comes out clean, then the cakes are ready.

Remove from the oven, turn out onto a rack to cool.

To decorate the cakes, cut a small cone shape into the top of each cake. Cut each cone in half to make two triangles. Spoon half a teaspoon of the strawberry jam and a teaspoon of the ricotta cream into the hole in the middle of each cake. Place the two triangles back on top of each cake at an angle to look like two butterfly wings. Sift the icing sugar over the top of the cakes and serve immediately.

For a food nerd: Replace the jam with berry compote (page 214).

1 **Serve:** 0.5g total fat • 0.1g saturated fat • 227kJ (54 calories) • 11g carbohydrates • 1g protein • 0.2g fibre

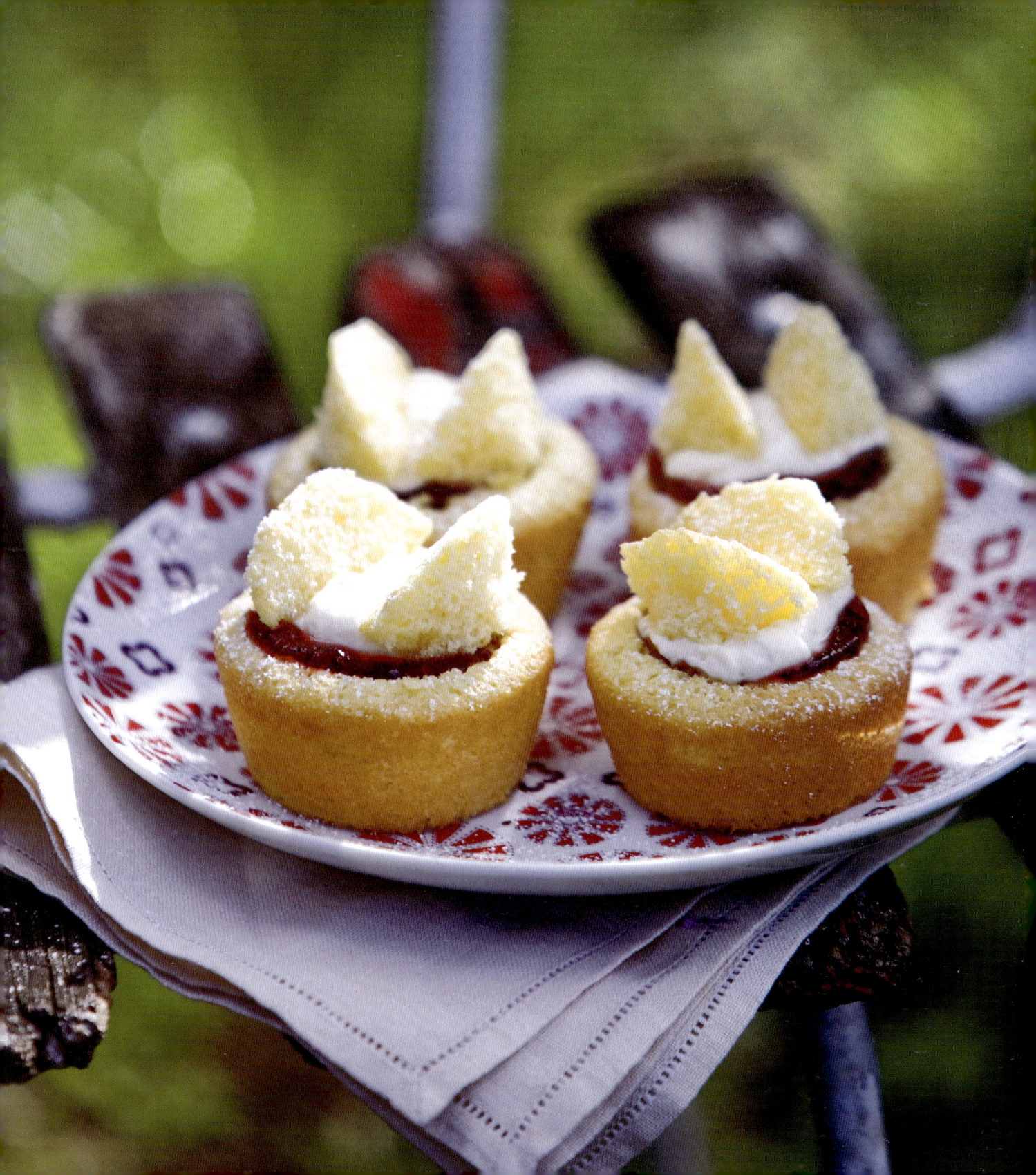

Banoffee Pie Towers

A banoffee pie is made from bananas, cream, pastry and a caramel toffee sauce and has a whopping 40 grams of fat per serve! Aside from the bananas, it is an incredibly indulgent dessert. The makeover uses a low-fat caramel toffee sauce, sponge finger biscuits in place of the pastry, lots of banana and ricotta cream in place of real cream. All of these are layered in a glass to create individual servings.

Serves: 4 • **Makes:** 4 towers • **Difficulty:** easy • **Takes:** 10 minutes to prep, 10 minutes to cook

4 sponge finger biscuits
5 ripe bananas, thinly sliced
1 quantity ricotta cream (page 217) or faux cream (page 217)

Caramel-toffee sauce
⅔ cup (160ml) light evaporated milk
3 teaspoons cornflour
2 heaped teaspoons brown sugar
2½ teaspoons golden syrup
2 teaspoons good quality spread

To make the sauce, mix 2 teaspoons of the evaporated milk with the cornflour to make a thin paste. Gently heat the rest of the milk (do not allow it to boil) and add the cornflour paste. Stir constantly as the sauce begins to thicken. Add the sugar, golden syrup and spread, and combine well. Heat for a further minute but do not cook any longer as it will continue to thicken as it cools. Remove from the heat and allow to cool.

To assemble the towers, break up the sponge fingers and divide half of them among four serving glasses.

Pour over some of the sauce, then spoon on some of the sliced banana. Next, place some of the ricotta cream or faux cream on top of the banana. Continue to layer each glass with the sponge fingers, sauce, bananas and ricotta or faux cream until finished.

Chill, then serve.

1 Serve: 2g total fat • 0.8g saturated fat • 1193kJ (284 calories) • 54g carbohydrates • 10g protein • 4g fibre

Strawberry Ricotta Tarts

These tarts have no pastry and are made with low-fat ricotta cheese, so they have all the delicacy of a tart but little of the fat.

Makes: 4 tarts • **Difficulty:** easy • **Takes:** 10 minutes to prep, 25 minutes to cook

good quality vegetable
oil cooking spray

1¼ cups (310g) low-fat
or extra-light ricotta
cheese

1 egg

2 teaspoons plain flour

2 tablespoons caster
sugar

4 strawberries, sliced

2 teaspoons strawberry
jam, warmed

Set the oven at 190°C.

With the cooking spray grease four muffin holes in a muffin pan.

Beat the ricotta, egg, flour and sugar with an electric mixer until smooth.

Spoon the mixture into the prepared muffin pan. Bake for 25 minutes until the tarts are just firm.

Allow to cool slightly, then remove from the pan and place on a serving plate. Arrange the sliced strawberries on top of each tart and gently paint the tarts (including the strawberry) with the warmed strawberry jam.

Serve.

For a food nerd: Use a mixture of berries in these, such as blueberries and raspberries.

1 **Serve:** 1g total fat • 0.4g saturated fat • 454kJ (108 calories) • 17g carbohydrates • 8g protein • 0.5g fibre

Truffles

These truffles are lovely and chocolatey but have only one tablespoon of cocoa powder, just fruit sugars for sweetness and next to no fat. They are a great sweet treat.

Makes: 35–40 truffles • **Difficulty:** easy • **Takes:** 10 minutes to prep

¾ cup (90g) sultanas
¾ cup (135g) seeded dates
1 tablespoon unsweetened
  cocoa powder
1 tablespoon boiling water
½ cup (125ml) skim milk
  powder
¼ cup (25g) almond meal
¼ cup (25g) desiccated coconut
4 tablespoons chocolate
  sprinkles or extra desiccated
  coconut for coating

Place the sultanas and dates in a food processor and blend until finely chopped. Add the cocoa powder, boiling water, skim milk powder, almond meal and coconut and pulse until just combined. The mixture should form a firm dough. Add a small amount of extra water if required to bring the dough together.

Take 1 teaspoon of mixture and roll into a ball. Repeat until all the mixture is used up. Toss the balls in the chocolate sprinkles or extra coconut to coat.

Store in an airtight container in the fridge for up to 2 weeks.

1 **Serve:** 1g total fat • 0.3g saturated fat • 143kJ (34 calories) • 6.2g carbohydrates • 0.6g protein • 0g fibre

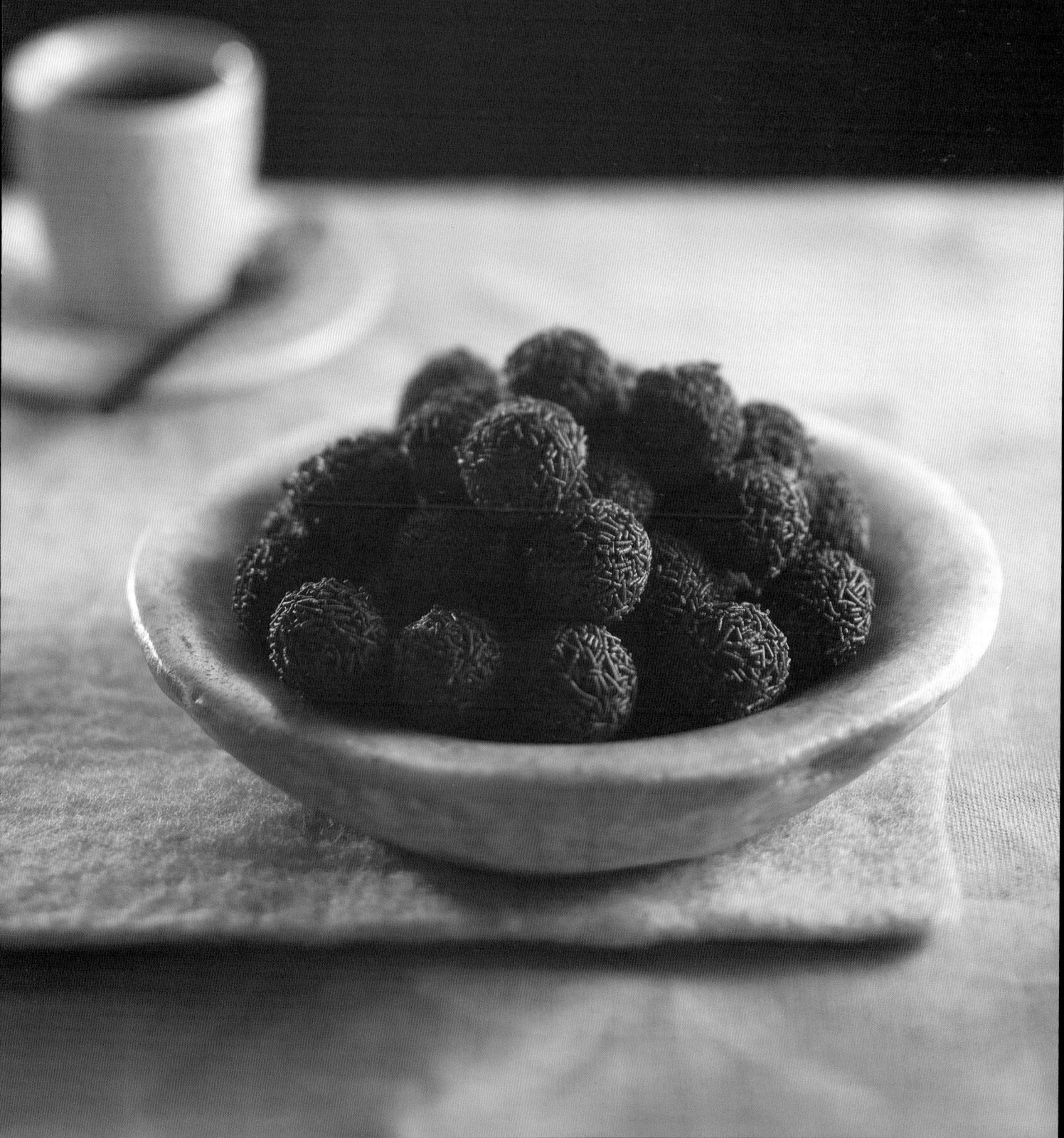

Lemon Tarts

Using reduced-fat pastry and only a small amount of reduced-fat spread in these tarts is a great improvement on the original lemon tart recipe. This recipe uses a gem baking pan. This looks like a normal muffin pan but the holes are shallow and rounded.

Makes: 24 tarts • **Difficulty:** medium • **Takes:** 15 minutes to prep, 15 minutes to cook

2 sheets 25% reduced-fat shortcrust pastry
¼ cup (30g) plain flour
¼ cup (30g) cornflour
¾ cup (165g) raw sugar
¾ cup (185ml) fresh lemon juice (2–3 lemons)
1½ tablespoons finely grated lemon zest
1¼ cups (310ml) water
4 egg yolks, lightly beaten
25g good quality spread, melted
1 tablespoon roughly chopped dark chocolate

Set the oven at 180°C.

On a lightly floured surface, roll out the pastry until 2mm thick. Using a 7–8cm scone cutter or glass, cut the pastry into 24 circles to fit two non-stick gem baking pans. Press the pastry into the moulds and blind bake for 15 minutes, or until just crisp. Set aside.

To make the lemon filling, place the flour, cornflour, sugar, lemon juice and zest in a small saucepan, and mix until well combined and smooth. Place over medium heat and gradually add the water, stirring constantly. Cook for 3–4 minutes, stirring constantly, until the mixture thickens. Remove from the heat and whisk in the egg yolks and the melted spread. Once completely combined, return to the heat and cook on very low heat for 3–4 minutes, or until very thick and glossy. Allow to cool for 5 minutes, then spoon the lemon filling into the cooked tart cases.

Melt the dark chocolate and, using a chopstick or knife, wave the melted chocolate over the tarts to drizzle thin stripes of chocolate on top.

1 Serve: 2g total fat • 1g saturated fat • 580kJ (138 calories) • 11g carbohydrates • 1g protein • 0.1g fibre

Chocolate Banana Cupcakes

Most cupcakes have around 125 grams of butter. This recipe uses only just over half that amount and replaces the butter with a healthier spread. The mashed banana lends flavour and also some of the moisture that is lost from having so little butter.

Makes: 24 cupcakes • **Difficulty:** easy • **Takes:** 15 minutes to prep, 15 minutes to cook

70g good quality spread

¼ cup (55g) raw sugar

1 egg, lightly beaten

1 tablespoon plum jam

½ ripe banana, chopped

⅓ cup (50g) wholemeal self-raising flour

⅓ cup (40g) self-raising flour

1 tablespoon unsweetened cocoa powder

¼ cup (60ml) low-fat evaporated milk, buttermilk or skim milk

Set the oven at 180°C.

Line a 12-hole muffin pan with paper cases.

Cream the spread and sugar until light and fluffy. Add the egg and mix until well combined. Add the jam and mix well. Then add the remaining ingredients and mix until just combined. Don't overbeat.

Spoon a tablespoon of the mixture into each of the paper cases. Bake for 15 minutes. Test if cooked by inserting a metal skewer in the middle of one of the cakes. If it comes out clean, then the cakes are ready.

1 Serve: 3g total fat • 0.5g saturated fat • 328kJ (78 calories) • 12g carbohydrates • 2g protein • 1g fibre

Profiteroles

These are tiny éclairs. They look and taste very French but their clever little differences to the originals make them a fab choice.

Makes: 14 mini profiteroles • **Difficulty:** medium • **Takes:** 10 minutes to prep, 30 minutes to cook

40g good quality spread
½ cup (125ml) water
½ cup (60g) plain flour
2 eggs
1 quantity ricotta cream
   (page 217) or cooled custard
   (page 213)
2 teaspoons icing sugar, to dust

Set the oven at 220°C.

Place the spread and water in a small saucepan and bring to the boil. Add the flour and stir vigorously with a wooden spoon until the mixture forms a smooth ball.

Transfer the ball to a small bowl and, using an electric mixer, beat in the eggs until the mixture is smooth and glossy. It will go crumbly and uneven while you are mixing. This is correct, continue mixing and, after a couple of minutes, the dough will come together.

Spoon the mixture into a piping bag or plastic bag with one tiny corner snipped off and pipe small dollops of the mixture onto baking-paper lined baking trays.

Place in the oven and bake for 8 minutes. Reduce the temperature to 180°C and bake for a further 8 minutes, or until the pastries are crisp.

Remove from the oven and make a small opening at the side of each pastry. Return to the oven and bake for a final 5 minutes. This will help to completely dry out the inside of the pastry. Set aside to cool.

Once cooled, gently cut the profiteroles open so that you can spoon some ricotta cream or chilled custard into the centre.

Dust with the icing sugar and serve.

1 Serve: 2g total fat • 0.4g saturated fat • 252kJ (60 calories) • 8g carbohydrates • 3g protein • 0.1g fibre

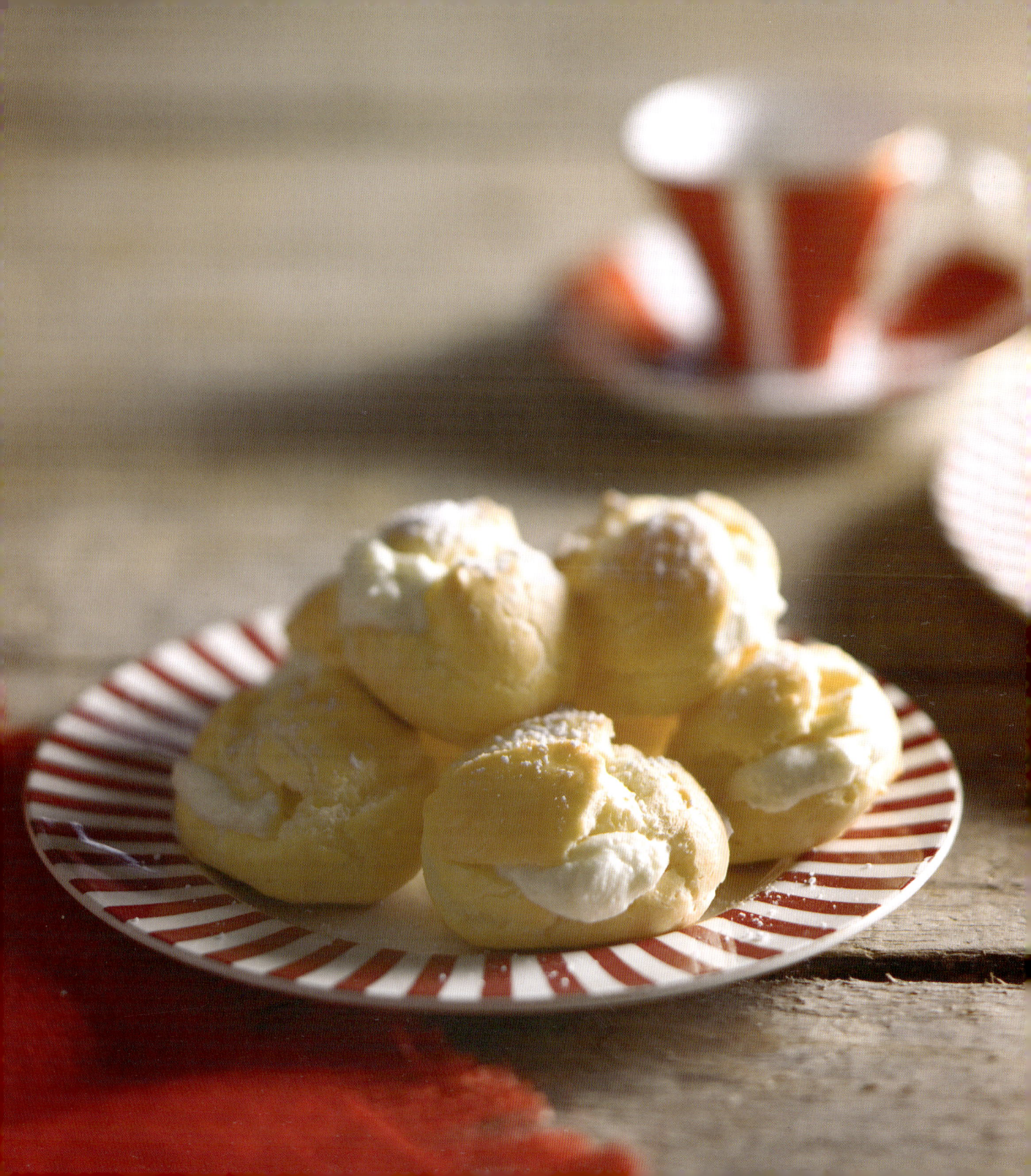

Apple Tea Cake

This is another afternoon tea treat which evokes strong childhood memories for many. Tea cakes are best eaten warm just after the cinnamon and sugar topping has been sprinkled on top. This cake is low in spread and sugar, and has the added bonus of including some apple.

Serves: 12 • **Makes:** 1 cake • **Difficulty:** easy • **Takes:** 10 minutes to prep, 50 minutes to cook

good quality cooking oil
  spray
90g good quality spread,
  softened
½ cup (110g) raw sugar
2 eggs, lightly beaten
¾ cup (90g) self-raising
  flour
¾ cup (110g) wholemeal
  self-raising flour
½ teaspoon baking
  powder
1 cup (200g) peeled and
  grated apple
⅓ cup (80ml) buttermilk
1 teaspoon extra of
  good quality spread
½ tablespoon caster
  sugar
½ teaspoon ground
  cinnamon

Set the oven at 180°C.

Spray and line a 20cm round cake tin.

Cream the spread and raw sugar until pale and fluffy. Add the eggs, one at a time, and mix in thoroughly. Stir in the flours, baking powder, apple and buttermilk, mixing well. Pour into the cake tin.

Bake in the oven for 50 minutes, or until cooked. Test if cooked by inserting a metal skewer in the middle of the cake. If it comes out clean, then the cake is ready.

Once removed from the oven, use a butter knife to spread the extra teaspoon of spread over the top of the warm cake.

Mix together the caster sugar and cinnamon and using a sifter sprinkle over the top of the cake.

For a food nerd: Add two tablespoons of wheat germ and don't peel the apple as there are lots of nutrients and fibre in and under the skin.

1 Serve: 4g total fat • 1g saturated fat • 567kJ (135 calories) • 22g carbohydrates • 3g protein • 0.5g fibre

Painkillers: the pain-free way to wean yourself from fat to fab

Making all the changes to take your diet from fat to fab means reducing fat, sugar and salt and boosting fibre and nutrients. It's not a diet as it's sustainable over the long term and will not interfere with your everyday routine once you are in the swing of it. You can use any of the fab recipes and tools in this book to adjust your current favourite recipes and to help you spot a new fab recipe when you are looking to expand your repertoire. No-one can survive on salad alone and why would we want to? This is about making your food fab so that you enjoy what you are eating.

The key is to do it slowly. Don't be too impatient and make all the changes at once, as this will inevitably set you up for failure. Your body and your family may well protest and withdraw their support if you make too many radical changes initially. Trust yourself to do it over a four- to five-week timeframe.

A pain-free Fat to Fab 5-week plan

Week 1: Reduce saturated fat (see page 15) and increase good fats like the essential fatty acids (see page 15).
Week 2: Boost nutrients and fibre (see pages 29 and 30).
Week 3: Cut down on sugar and work on stress management (see pages 25 and 125).
Week 4: Adjust portion size (see page 202).
Week 5: Cut down on salt and become an expert label reader (see pages 29 and 78).

For more detailed menu plans, have a look at page 236–239 in Resources.

Vanilla Slice

It is easy to give vanilla slice a makeover by using a homemade low-fat, thick custard and reduced-fat pastry. Often vanilla slice is iced, but this version is sweet enough without the icing and just needs a light dusting of icing sugar to finish it off before serving. This fab version has only one-fifth of the fat of the traditional slice.

Makes: 9 pieces • **Difficulty:** medium • **Takes:** 30 minutes to prep, 10 minutes to cook

2 sheets 25% reduced-fat
   puff pastry, thawed
1 teaspoon icing sugar,
   for dusting

Custard filling

3 egg yolks
2¼ cups (560ml) skim milk
   or low-fat evaporated
   milk
4½ tablespoons honey or
   raw sugar
3½ tablespoons plain
   flour
1 teaspoon natural vanilla
   extract

Line a 23cm square cake tin with baking paper.

To make the filling, beat the egg yolks until thick and pale in colour. Set aside. Heat the milk until it just begins to foam. Immediately remove from the stove and set aside. Working quickly, add the honey or sugar and flour to the egg yolks and mix well. Stirring constantly, add 2 tablespoons of the hot milk to the egg mixture. While continually stirring, gradually add all of the milk to the eggs and stir until combined.

Pour the egg and milk mixture back into the saucepan and place over medium heat. Stir constantly until it thickens. It will continue to thicken when it cools. Whisk in the vanilla.

Pass the filling through a sieve if there are any lumps. Set aside to cool.

Roll out each sheet of thawed pastry to 3mm thick and place on a baking-paper lined baking tray. Prick the pastry all over with a fork. Place in the oven and bake for 8–10 minutes, or until golden.

Trim each cooked sheet of pastry to form a 23cm square and place one sheet on the bottom of the prepared cake tin.

Spoon the cooled filling onto the pastry base and spread evenly. Place a second sheet of pastry on top of the custard. Refrigerate for at least an hour.

When serving, dust with the icing sugar and cut carefully into squares with a serrated knife.

1 Serve: 3.3g total fat • 1.5g saturated fat • 1268kJ (302 calories) • 20g carbohydrates • 4g protein • 0.1g fibre

Matchsticks

This old-fashioned treat, sometimes called mille-feuille, is two layers of pastry, often smeared with jam and filled with imitation or fresh cream. The recipe below reduces the fat from 22 grams to just 2 grams, improves the flavour and increases the real fruit content.

Serves: 4 • **Makes:** 4 matchsticks • **Difficulty:** easy • **Takes:** 10 minutes to prep, 10 minutes to cook

½ sheet 25% reduced-fat puff pastry, thawed

1 cup (170g) frozen mixed berries (not strawberries)

3 teaspoons sugar

1½ teaspoon cornflour

4 teaspoons water

1 teaspoon icing sugar, to dust

1 quantity faux cream (page 217), ricotta cream (page 217) or ⅓ cup (80ml) low-fat vanilla yoghurt

Set the oven at 180°C.

Cut the puff pastry sheet into 4 rectangles (each approximately 6 x 12cm). Place the rectangles on a baking-paper lined baking tray and bake for 8–10 minutes, or until the pastry is lightly browned and crisp. Remove and allow to cool.

Meanwhile, in a small saucepan, combine the berries and the sugar. Place over medium heat and simmer until the berries begin to thaw and the juices run.

In a small bowl, mix together the water and cornflour to make a smooth paste. Add the paste to the berry mixture and simmer until the sauce thickens and turns clear (this means the cornflour is cooked), stirring occasionally. Allow to cool.

Carefully pull each pastry rectangle apart to make eight thin pastry rectangles.

On four of the rectangles, spread some of the faux or ricotta cream, or yoghurt then add a tablespoon of the berry compote. Place a pastry rectangle on top.

Sift the icing sugar on top of the matchstick and serve immediately.

For a food nerd: Serve without the pastry lid. It tastes just as yummy, looks beautiful with the berries on top and halves the fat from the pastry.

1 Serve: 2g total fat • 1g saturated fat • 395kJ (94 calories) • 18g carbohydrates • 6g protein • 2g fibre

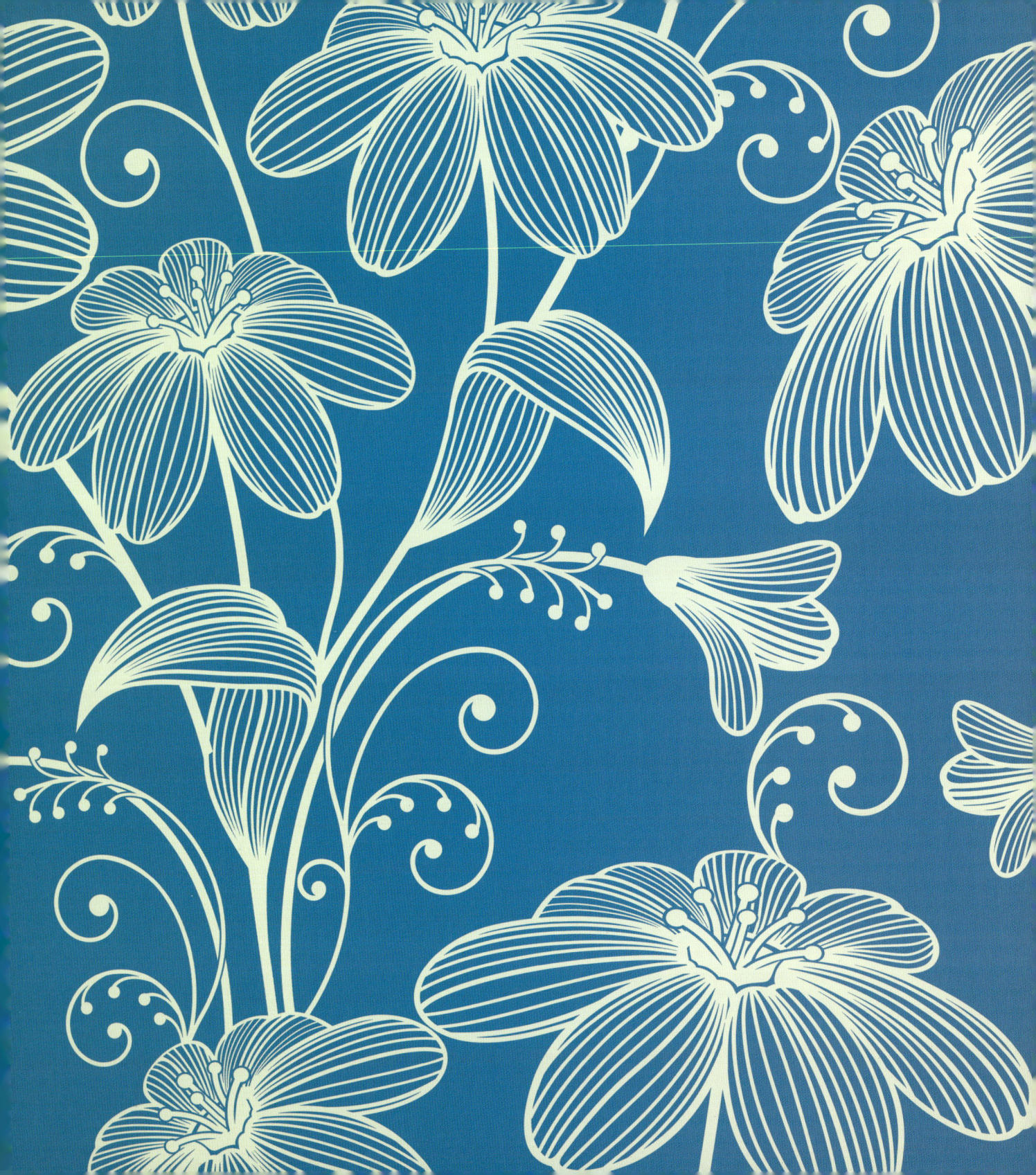

Dinner

Creamy pastas and curries, fatty roasts, oily Asian dishes, cheesy Italian favourites all make it onto the fat list for dinners. You are sure to find your fat favourites among this selection of dinner recipes. If not, adapt them using the tricks and tools used to whip these dinner recipes into shape.

Use a selection of these fab dishes to throw a dinner party for eight or perhaps a romantic evening or two.

Dinner party for eight
Cream of pumpkin soup (page 66)

Creamy marinara (page 130)

Rocket, pear and pea salad (page 158)

Caprese salad (page 170)

Pear crumble (page 199)

Romantic evening for two
Garlic prawns (page 128)

Fettuccine carbonara (page 142)

Watercress, parsley and beetroot salad

Crispy Cajun Chicken

This is spicy fried chicken minus the fat. If you like it extra spicy, double the Cajun seasoning to a full teaspoon.

Serves: 4 • **Difficulty:** easy • **Takes:** 10 minutes to prep, 20 minutes to cook

⅓ cup (40g) plain flour

2 eggs, whisked

2 tablespoons finely chopped flat-leaf parsley

1 cup (100g) fine breadcrumbs

½ teaspoon Cajun seasoning

¼ teaspoon garlic powder

¼ teaspoon onion powder

8 drumsticks, skin removed or 3 large (400g) skinless chicken breast fillets

olive oil cooking spray

Set the oven at 210°C.

Place the flour in a bowl.

Mix the whisked eggs and parsley in a second bowl.

Mix the breadcrumbs, Cajun seasoning, garlic powder and onion powder in a third bowl.

Coat the drumsticks in the flour, then the egg and parsley mix and finally the breadcrumb mix. If using chicken breast, cut into 2cm thick diagonal slices (escalopes) and then coat as for the drumsticks. Refrigerate for 20 minutes.

Line a baking tray with baking paper. Spread the chicken out on the tray and spray with the cooking oil.

For the drumsticks: Place in the oven for 20 minutes, then turn and bake for another 10–15 minutes, or until there is no pink flesh and the drumsticks are cooked through.

For the chicken breast: Place in the oven for 6 minutes, then turn and bake for another 6 minutes, or until just cooked through.

Serving suggestion: Serve with cucumber raita (page 169) and harissa rice salad (page 172).

1 Serve: 3.7g total fat • 1g saturated fat • 878kJ (209 calories) • 7g carbohydrates • 27g protein • 0.1g fibre

Wiener Schnitzel

Here, you bake the schnitzel in the oven so it becomes crispy, bypassing the deep-fryer.

Serves: 4 • **Difficulty:** easy • **Takes:** 30 minutes to prep (including fridge time), 15 minutes to cook

1 cup (125g) plain flour
1 egg white, beaten
1½ cups (100g)
  breadcrumbs
¼ cup finely chopped
  flat-leaf parsley
400g lean veal escalopes
olive oil cooking spray
4 lemon wedges, to
  serve

Set the oven at 200°C.

Place the flour in a bowl, and the egg white in another bowl.

In a third bowl, combine the breadcrumbs with the parsley.

Using a meat mallet, gently pound the escalopes until 5mm thick.

Dip the veal in the flour, then in the egg white and finally coat with the parsley breadcrumbs. Place in the fridge for 20 minutes.

Line a baking tray with baking paper and spray with the oil.

Remove the veal from the fridge and place on the baking tray. Spray the veal with the oil. Place in the oven for 10 minutes, then turn the meat over and reduce the temperature to 180°C. Cook for a further 5 minutes, or until the meat is cooked through.

Serve with the lemon wedges.

Serving suggestion: Serve with a fresh red or green salsa (pages 164 and 165) and a rainbow salad (page 166) with at least four different vegetables.

For a food nerd: Serve with good quality sauerkraut, which is excellent for digestive health.

1 Serve: 8g total fat • 2.5g saturated fat • 1569kJ (373.5 calories) • 21g carbohydrates • 38g protein • 0.1g fibre

Chicken Parmigiana

Traditional parmigiana drips with cheese and oil. This version cuts down on the cheese and oil and uses the oven instead of the frying pan to get the desired result.

Serves: 4 • **Difficulty:** easy • **Takes:** 30 minutes to prep (including fridge time), 15 minutes to cook

⅔ cup (65g) breadcrumbs

2 teaspoons finely chopped oregano (or 1 teaspoon dried)

1 egg, whisked

2 large (400g) skinless chicken breast fillets

olive oil cooking spray

Sauce

2 teaspoons extra virgin olive oil

½ brown or red onion, diced

1 clove garlic, crushed

½ zucchini, grated

200g tinned tomatoes

1 tablespoon tomato paste

1 teaspoon finely chopped oregano (or ½ teaspoon dried)

Set the oven at 200°C.

Place the whisked egg in a bowl. In another small bowl, mix the breadcrumbs with the oregano.

Slice the chicken lengthways into four 5mm thick steaks. Coat each chicken piece first in the egg and then in the breadcrumbs and oregano. Place in the fridge for 20 minutes.

Line a baking tray with baking paper and spray with the oil.

Remove the chicken from the fridge and place on the baking tray. Spray the chicken with the oil and then place in the oven for 10 minutes. Turn the chicken over, and reduce the temperature to 180°C and cook for a further 5 minutes, or until the chicken is just cooked through.

Meanwhile, make the sauce by heating the oil in a saucepan over medium heat. Add the onion and garlic and lightly fry for 2–3 minutes, or until soft. Add the zucchini and cook for a further 2–3 minutes or until just translucent. Add the tinned tomatoes, tomato paste, oregano, thyme, fresh tomato, salt, sugar and pepper. Cook for a further 5 minutes on a low simmer. Add the basil. Cook for a further 3 minutes, and then remove from heat.

1 teaspoon finely
   chopped thyme (or
   ½ teaspoon dried)
1 tomato, finely diced
pinch each of salt and raw
   sugar
3 grinds of pepper
4 basil leaves, finely
   shredded (optional)
2 tablespoons low-fat
   finely grated mozzarella
   cheese

Place the 4 chicken pieces on 4 heat-proof serving plates.

Spoon 1–1½ tablespoons of the sauce over each piece of chicken and finish with the grated mozzarella cheese. Return the chicken to the oven and bake for 5 minutes until the cheese is melted.

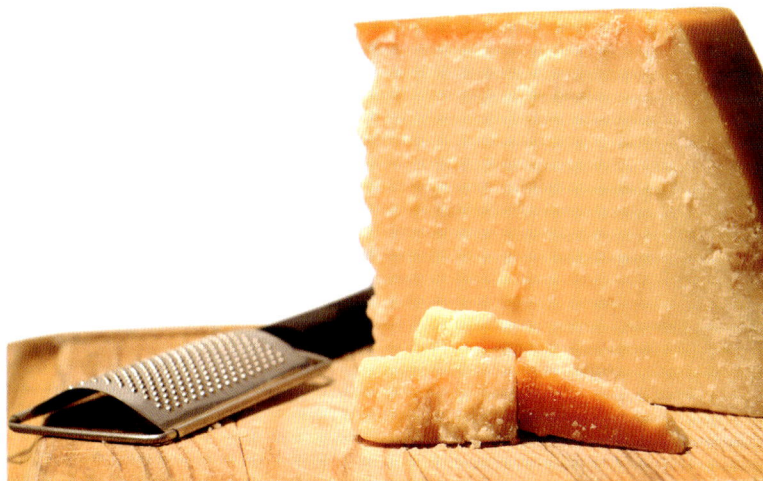

Serving suggestion: Serve with a rainbow salad (page 166).

For a food nerd: Serve with mixed steamed vegetables.

1 Serve: 5.6g total fat • 1.5g saturated fat • 890kJ (212 calories) • 8g carbohydrates • 27g protein • 1.4g fibre

Green Chicken Curry

Like red curry paste, green curry paste varies considerably between brands so check labels very carefully. Look at the total fat and saturated fat content. A serve of this fab curry is only 5.5 grams of fat. The fat version has 66 grams!

Serves: 4 • **Difficulty:** medium • **Takes:** 20 minutes to prep, 25 minutes to cook

1 teaspoon peanut oil

500g skinless chicken breast fillets, fat trimmed and sliced into chunks

1½ tablespoons low-fat green curry paste

2 fresh kaffir lime leaves, spines removed and roughly chopped

1 tablespoon brown sugar

2 tablespoons fish sauce

¼ cup chopped Thai or sweet basil leaves

¼ cup chopped coriander

250g green beans, trimmed and sliced into 3cm pieces

2 zucchini, finely sliced

½ cup (125ml) water

2 cups (500ml) low-fat coconut-flavoured evaporated milk

12 snow peas, trimmed

2 tablespoons flat-leaf parsley leaves

1 long green chilli, thinly sliced

2 spring onions thinly sliced

Heat the peanut oil in a large frying pan to medium-hot and cook the chicken in batches, until just cooked through. Remove from the pan and drain on absorbent paper.

Fry the curry paste in the pan for 1–2 minutes until fragrant. Add the lime leaves. Cook for a further minute, stirring constantly.

Add the sugar, fish sauce, Thai basil, coriander, green beans, zucchini and water to the curry mixture and stir to combine. Cook for 5 minutes, or until the vegetables are just tender.

Add the evaporated milk, chicken and snow peas, and simmer for a further 2 minutes until the milk, chicken and the snow peas are gently warmed through.

Serve topped with parsley, chilli and spring onions.

Serving suggestion: Serve with brown rice and lightly steamed broccoli and cauliflower.

For a food nerd: Replace the chicken with a 400g tin of drained and washed chickpeas.

1 Serve: 5.5g total fat • 2.2g saturated fat • 1451kJ (345.5 calories) • 32g carbohydrates • 42g protein • 4g fibre

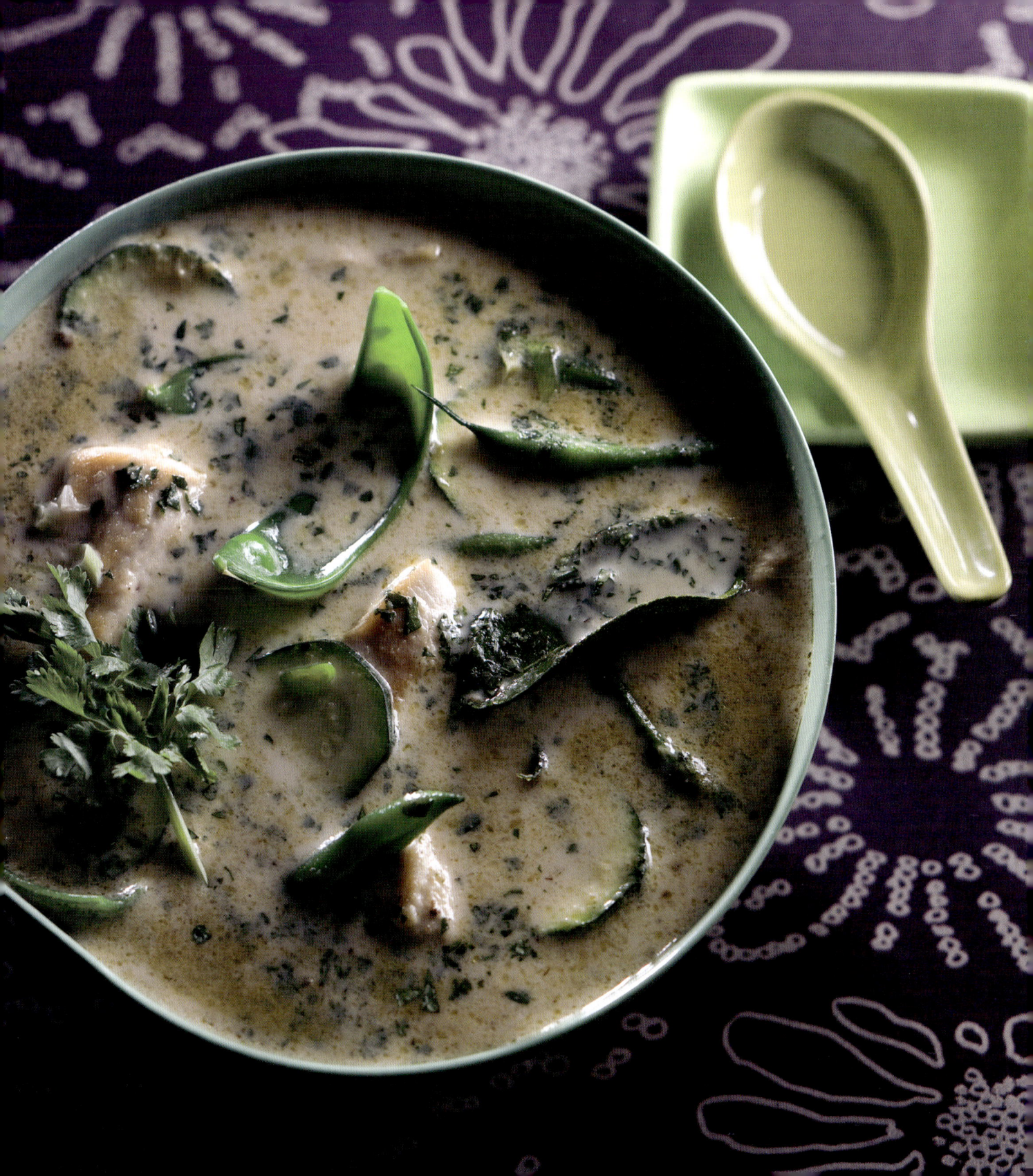

Creamy Chicken Risotto

Risotto is usually fine nutritionally until the end when butter and cheese are added and, sometimes, cream. They give it a smooth, creamy texture but using low-fat evaporated milk gives the same effect without the fat. The consistency should be a little like a rice pudding, as the rice should not absorb all of the liquid. Add a small amount of stock if it starts to become gluggy.

Serves: 6 • **Difficulty:** easy • **Takes:** 10 minutes to prep, 25 minutes to cook

2 teaspoons extra virgin
  olive oil
6 shallots, thinly sliced
400g skinless chicken
  breast fillets, cut into
  thin strips
2 cups (440g) arborio rice
1½ litres chicken stock
1 cup (250ml) low-fat
  evaporated milk
zest of 1 small lemon
1 cup (155g) frozen peas
2 cups (120g) broccoli
  florets
2 corn cobs, kernels sliced
  from cobs
2 tablespoons finely
  chopped chives
2 teaspoons finely
  chopped tarragon
2 tablespoons finely
  chopped flat-leaf
  parsley

Heat the oil in a large heavy-based saucepan over medium-hot heat. Fry the shallots until soft, then add the chicken and cook until the chicken just begins to brown.

Turn down the heat and add the rice, stock, evaporated milk and lemon zest. Simmer, uncovered, over low-medium heat for 20 minutes, stirring regularly, until the rice is soft but there is still enough liquid that the rice is not gluggy. Add a small amount of stock if more liquid is required.

Add the peas, broccoli, corn, chives, tarragon and parsley and combine well. Cook, covered, for a further 5 minutes, stirring occasionally, or until the vegetables are just tender.

Serve immediately.

Serving suggestion: Serve with caprese salad (page 170).

For a food nerd: Boost up the vegetables by adding mushrooms, grated zucchini and pumpkin.

1 **Serve:** 3.5g total fat • 1g saturated fat • 1672kJ (398 calories) • 66g carbohydrates • 26g protein • 3.4g fibre

Thai Fish Cakes

Thai fish cakes make it onto the fat list as they are deep-fried. This lightly pan-fried version is much lower in fat and will knock your socks off.

Serves: 4 • **Makes:** 8 fishcakes • **Difficulty:** medium • **Takes:** 10 minutes to prep, 1 hour in fridge, 10 minutes to cook

500g ling, basa or white boneless fish fillet, roughly chopped

2 tablespoons low-fat red curry paste

1 tablespoon fish sauce

1 egg

½ teaspoon sugar

12 round beans, trimmed and thinly sliced

3 kaffir lime leaves, spine removed, finely shredded

1 tablespoon extra virgin olive oil

Dipping Sauce

½ cup cold water

¼ cup (60ml) white vinegar

⅓ cup (75g) sugar

1 teaspoon Lebanese cucumber, deseeded, finely chopped

½ long red chilli, deseeded, finely chopped

2 teaspoons fish sauce

To make the dipping sauce, combine the cold water, vinegar and sugar in a small saucepan over low heat. Cook for 4 minutes, stirring until the sugar is dissolved. Bring to a simmer and cook for a further 5 minutes, or until it thickens to a runny syrup. Remove from heat. Combine with the cucumber, chilli and fish sauce. Leave to cool.

For the fish cakes, place the fish, curry paste, fish sauce, egg and sugar in a food processor, and pulse until just combined. In a small bowl, mix together the beans, kaffir lime leaves and the fish mixture. Stir until well combined. Cover and refrigerate for 1 hour.

Remove from the fridge and, with wet hands, shape tablespoons of the mixture into balls and then gently flatten into patties.

Heat the oil on a hot griddle pan and cook the fish cakes in batches until browned and cooked through (3–4 minutes on each side, depending on the thickness of the cakes).

Serve with the dipping sauce.

Serving suggestion: Serve with potato salad (page 171) and a green salad.

1 Serve: 5.4g total fat • 1.4g saturated fat • 302kJ (72 calories) • 4g carbohydrates • 2g protein • 0.6g fibre

Singapore Noodles

Singapore noodles are filled with cheap, fatty meat and fried in lots of oil. The oil has been cut here and the bacon is as lean as possible. It makes no difference to the taste, but it makes a big difference to the healthiness of it. When buying packet noodles, always check the ingredients label to ensure they are preservative free and have no additives.

Serves: 4 • **Difficulty:** easy • **Takes:** 15 minutes to prep, 10 minutes to cook

440g fresh Singapore noodles
  or egg noodles
2 teaspoons peanut oil
1 brown onion, finely sliced
1 rasher 97% fat-free bacon,
  diced
3cm piece fresh ginger, grated
1 carrot, cut into matchsticks
300g skinless chicken breast
  fillets, sliced into thin strips
1 tablespoon curry powder
  (1½ for mild-hot)
1 cup bean shoots, tails removed
4 spring onions, thinly sliced
1½ tablespoons tamari or light
  soy sauce
⅓ cup (80ml) sweet sherry or
  Chinese cooking wine

Prepare the noodles as per the directions on the packet. Drain.

Heat the oil in a wok and add the onion, bacon, ginger, carrot and chicken and stir-fry until the chicken is just cooked through. Add the curry powder and cook for a further 1 minute to release the flavours.

Add the noodles and the remaining ingredients to the pan, and stir-fry for a further 5 minutes.

Serve.

For a food nerd: Use dried rice vermicelli, soaked in boiling water, for grain variation and less preservatives.

1 Serve: 6.6g total fat • 1g saturated fat • 1356kJ (323 calories) • 41g carbohydrates • 25.5g protein • 2g fibre

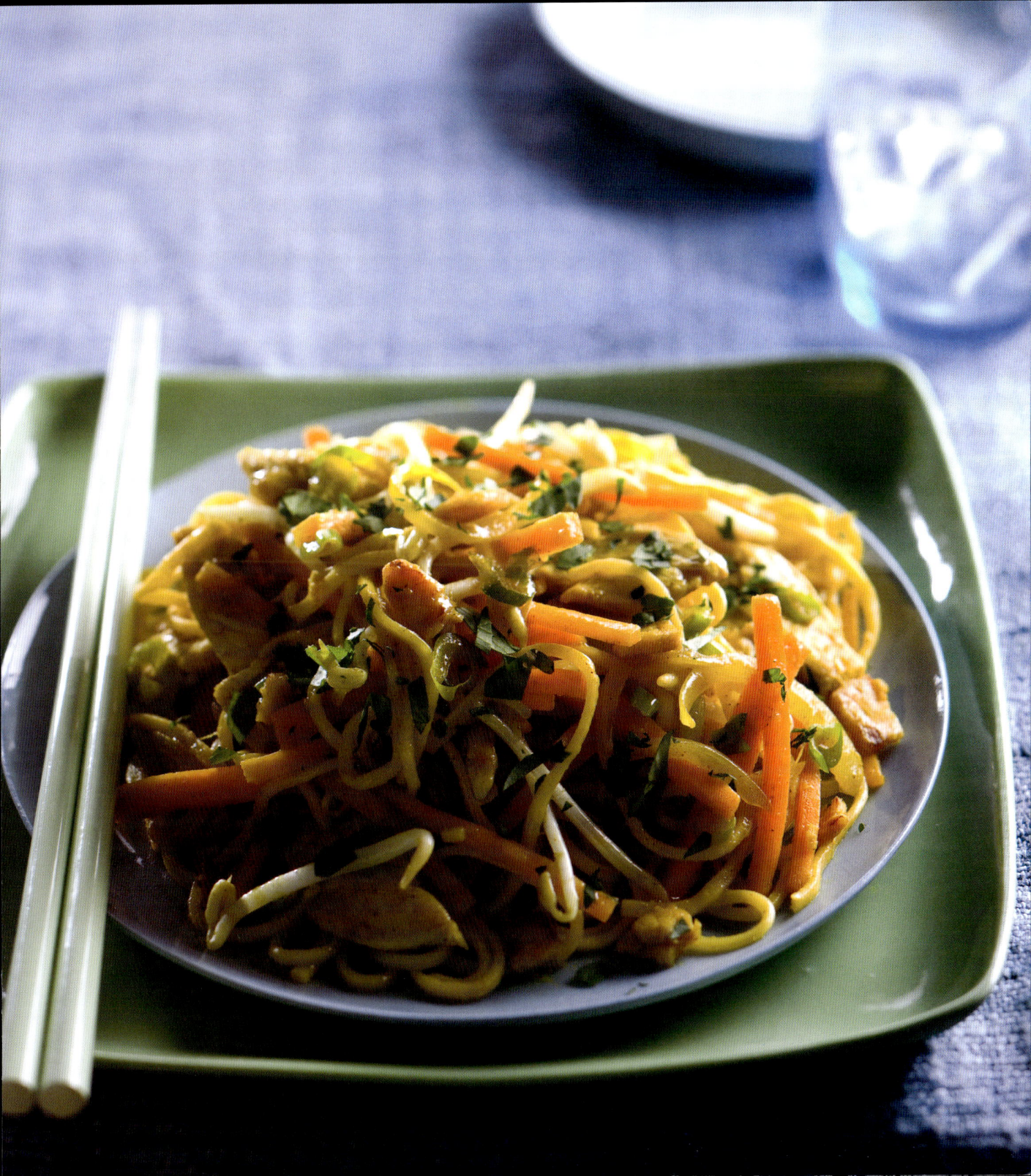

Chilli Con Carne

This recipe has been made over by using lean, good quality minced meat and very little oil. The flavour comes from the spices and the simmering time rather than lots of salt and oil.

When using minced beef pay a little bit more and buy organic. It is not much more expensive than conventional mince, but, being organic, is guaranteed to be free from all pesticides, hormones and antibiotics.

Serves: 4 • **Difficulty:** easy • **Takes:** 15 minutes to prep, 20 minutes to cook

olive oil cooking spray
2 brown onions, sliced
2 cloves garlic, crushed
1 green capsicum, diced
300g extra lean organic minced beef
½ teaspoon chilli powder
1 small red chilli, deseeded and finely diced
1 teaspoon hot paprika
2 tablespoons tomato paste
2 x 400g tins diced tomatoes
pinch of salt
400g tin red kidney beans

Spray a heavy-based saucepan with the oil and heat to medium-hot. Add the onions and garlic and cook until soft. Stir in the capsicum and meat, cook until the meat is browned. Add the chilli powder, chilli, paprika, tomato paste, tinned tomatoes and salt. Bring to the boil, then reduce heat to low and simmer for 15–20 minutes, uncovered, stirring occasionally. Add the kidney beans and cook for a further 5 minutes, or until the beans are warmed through.

Serve.

Serving suggestion: Serve with a mixed green leaf salad.

For a food nerd: Thicken this sauce with a mix of pureed vegetables. For a vegetarian version, omit the meat, add some four bean mix and 2 cups of mixed, diced vegetables.

1 **Serve:** 13.4g total fat • 5.2g saturated fat • 1411kJ (336 calories) • 31g carbohydrates • 23g protein • 8g fibre

Stress – the saboteur

Stress is an ongoing symptom of the frantic modern lifestyle most of us lead and is the cause of more than three absent work days a year for every worker.

Stress affects the nerves that run between our brain and digestive system, which is why stress can have such a marked impact on our digestion. For example, stress can slow digestion, cause pain, bloating or changes in bowel habits and, in the longer term, cause more serious illnesses and dysfunction. In fact, 95% of the body's serotonin, a hormone that manages mood, is found in the digestive system, not the brain. We can eat the world's healthiest diet but if we are not digesting it well, we will not enjoy any benefits from our hard work.

By making some small diet and lifestyle changes, you can ensure that you better cope with the stresses in your life and keep your healthy eating goals on track.

1. Eat foods rich in vitamin C, the B vitamins and antioxidants.
Stress can quickly deplete your stores of many vitamins and minerals, such as the B vitamins and vitamin C. Stress-busting foods include wheat germ, pecans, sunflower seeds, almonds, berries, capsicum, blackcurrants, broccoli, guava, watercress, kale, grapefruit, oranges and strawberries.

2. Limit your intake of processed foods and stimulants.
Pre-prepared and packaged foods, white flour products, white sugar and caffeine drinks (coffee, tea, cola) can exacerbate the effects of stress.

3. Practise good eating discipline
How you are eating is just as important as *what* you are eating. Take five deep breaths before you eat to relax your shoulders and stimulate the parasympathetic nervous system, the calming side of your nervous system which controls digestion. Then clear your mind, bring yourself into the present, and take at least 15 minutes to eat your meal. Smell and savour the food, chew well and sit for five minutes after the meal to allow it to begin digesting. No matter how busy you are, 20 minutes will not break the bank but it will make a huge difference to your wellbeing and how you digest your food.

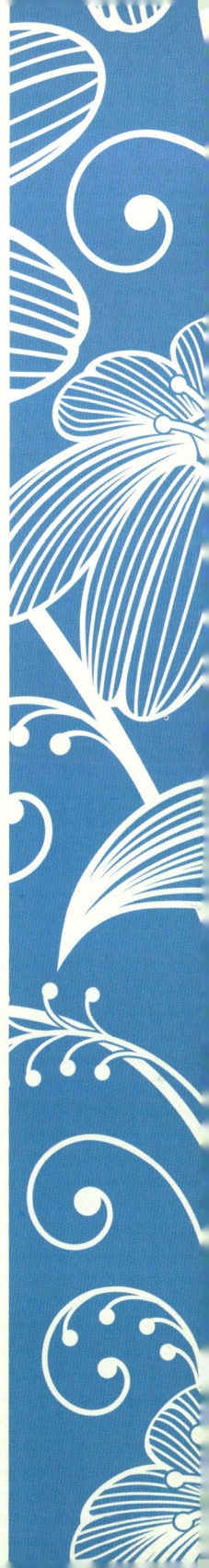

Fish and Chips

Most of us, when being honest, feel pretty awful after a heavy, deep-fried meal like traditional fish and chips and it's no surprise that it comes in at over 50 grams of fat. It is the ultimate fat meal but can be easily made over to still taste delicious and be healthier, leaving us feeling a whole lot better.

Serves: 4 • **Difficulty:** easy • **Takes:** 15 minutes to prep, 20 minutes to cook

olive oil cooking spray
1 egg white, beaten
zest of 1 lemon
1 tablespoon chopped parsley
⅔ cup (65g) breadcrumbs
4 flathead, bream, basa or ling fillets, skinned and bones removed
double batch of chips (page 74)
low-fat tartare sauce, to serve

Set the oven at 200°C.

Line a baking tray with baking paper and spray with the oil.

In a bowl place the egg white. In a separate bowl mix the lemon zest with the parsley and breadcrumbs.

Coat the fish with the egg white and then with the breadcrumbs. Place on the lined tray and spray the top of the fillets with the oil. Cook for 5–10 minutes depending on the size and thickness of the fillets.

Serve with the chips and a tablespoon of low-fat tartare sauce.

Serving suggestion: Serve with a rainbow salad (page 166) or coleslaw (page 160).

For a food nerd: Replace the tartare sauce with a spicy salsa (pages 164 and 165).

1 Serve: 6g total fat • 1g saturated fat • 1970kJ (469 calories) • 74g carbohydrates • 25.5g protein • 9.4g fibre

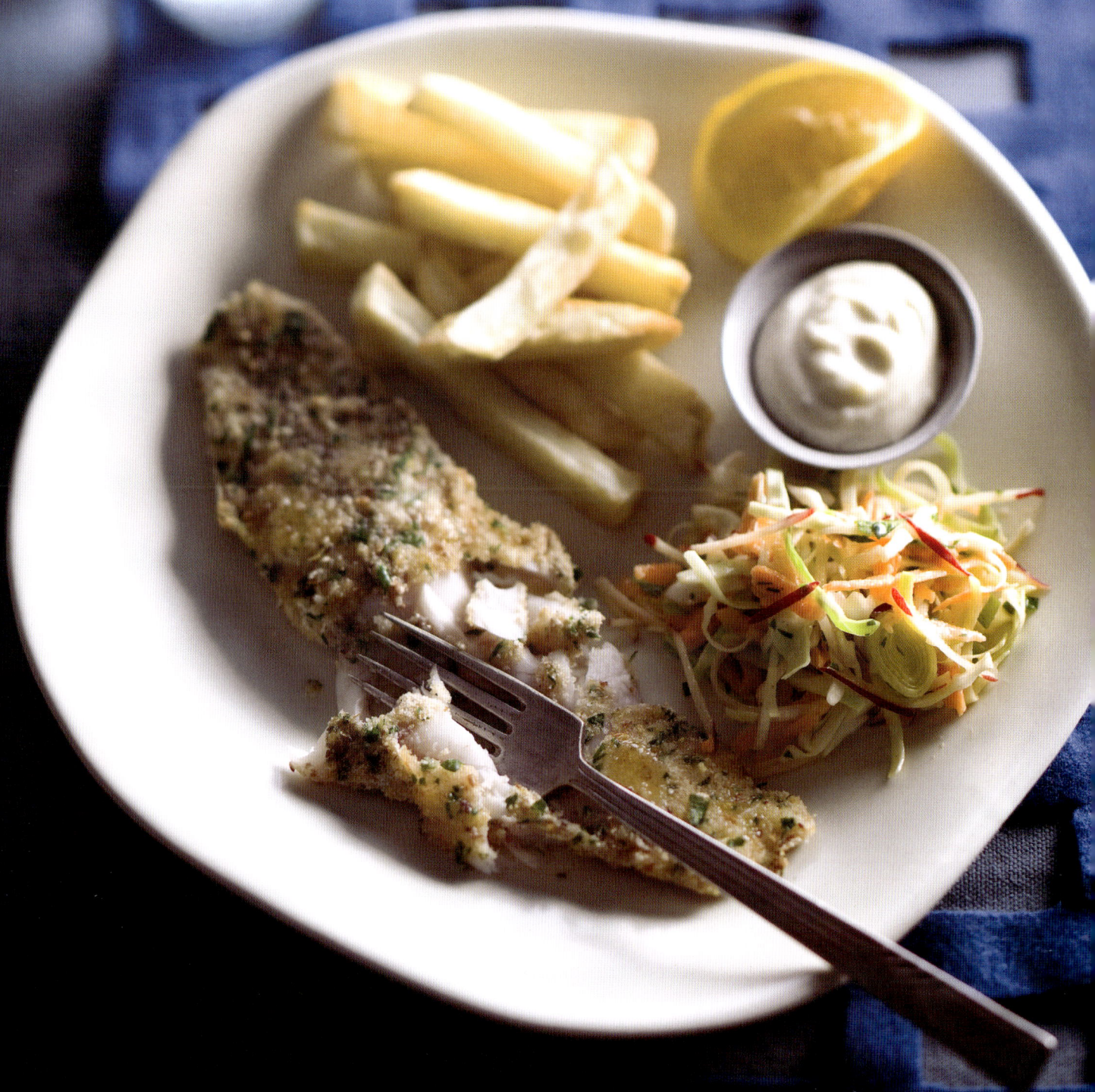

Garlic Prawns

Traditional garlic prawns are baked and served in an oil and butter bath. This recipe uses white wine, stock and lemon juice with the garlic to pack a flavour punch while keeping it lean and healthy.

Serves: 4 • **Difficulty**: medium • **Takes**: 10 minutes to prep (overnight to marinade), 10 minutes to cook

8 cloves garlic, finely chopped

pinch of salt

¼ teaspoon pepper

1 tablespoon extra virgin olive oil

24 green prawns, peeled and deveined

⅓ cup (80ml) white wine

⅓ cup (80ml) vegetable stock

1 tablespoon lemon juice

¼ cup (15g) chopped flat-leaf parsley

The day before, prepare the prawn marinade by combining the garlic, salt, pepper and oil in a bowl. Toss the prawns in the marinade, coating them well. Cover and refrigerate overnight to allow the flavours to develop.

Set the oven at 220°C.

Remove the prawns from the marinade and arrange them in a single layer in four individual ramekins or ovenproof dishes.

Add the white wine, vegetable stock and lemon juice to the marinade. Stir together and then pour equal amounts into the four dishes.

Cover the dishes with lids or foil and bake for 10 minutes, or until the prawns are just cooked (that is when the flesh has just turned white).

Sprinkle with the parsley to serve.

Serving suggestion: Serve with a garden salad.

For a food nerd: Serve with a bitter green salad (rocket, mizuna, watercress leaves) and a caprese salad (page 170).

1 Serve: 3.7g total fat • 0.6g saturated fat • 344kJ (82 calories) • 3g carbohydrates • 9.3g protein • 0.4g fibre

Creamy Tuna Mornay

With a reduction in cheese, cream and other full-fat dairy, you can significantly trim down tuna mornay without losing the signature creamy taste. Use low-fat milk or, for an even creamier finish, opt for low-fat evaporated milk. If you are looking to feed a large family with high energy needs, cook 2 cups of wholemeal small pasta shells and stir them through the mornay before serving.

Serves: 4 • **Difficulty:** easy • **Takes:** 30 minutes to prep, 15 minutes to cook

2 corn cobs

2 tablespoons good
quality spread

3½ tablespoons plain flour

1 white onion, finely diced

¼ teaspoon pepper

375ml tin low-fat
evaporated milk

½ cup (125ml) skim milk

425g tin tuna in
spingwater, drained and
flaked

½ cup tasty low-fat grated
cheese

1 tablespoon chopped
flat-leaf parsley

Steam the corn until tender. Set aside to cool.

In a medium sized saucepan, melt the spread. Add the flour and stir to combine. This is a roux that is the basis of a white or mornay sauce. Cook the roux for 1 minute to ensure the flour is cooked through. Add the onion and cook for a further minute. Add the pepper.

Remove from heat and slowly add the milks, stirring all the time. Place back over medium heat, stirring constantly until the sauce is smooth and thick. Remove from heat.

When cool, cut the corn kernels from the cob.

Add the tuna, corn and cheese to the mornay sauce and stir to combine. Place over medium heat and stir until warmed through.

Serve sprinked with the parsley.

Serving suggestion: Serve with a leafy green salad.

For a food nerd: Replace 1 cup (250ml) of the milk with low-salt vegetable stock or, if you do not eat any dairy, use low-fat soy milk and stock.

1 Serve: 6.7g total fat • 2.8g saturated fat • 1348kJ (321 calories) • 24.5g carbohydrates • 33g protein • 0g fibre

Creamy Marinara

You won't believe this creamy sauce has no actual cream in it. The blend of flavours in this delicate sauce is delightful and complements the seafood. It has some wine in it, but all the alcohol (and kilojoules) will be carried off in the steam when you simmer it.

Serves: 4 • **Difficulty:** medium • **Takes:** 30 minutes to prep, 15 minutes to cook

300g spaghetti

2 cloves garlic, crushed

½ cup (125ml) vegetable stock

1 shallot, finely sliced

⅓ cup (80ml) dry white wine

1 cup (250ml) low-fat evaporated milk

2 teaspoons cornflour

2 tablespoons finely grated lemon zest

pinch of salt

pinch of white pepper

700g fresh marinara mix

2 teaspoons extra virgin olive oil

1 tablespoon finely chopped flat-leaf parsley

1 tablespoon finely chopped dill

Cook the spaghetti according to the directions on the packet. Drain Well.

Meanwhile, in a saucepan, combine the garlic, stock, shallot and white wine. Bring to the boil, then reduce heat to low and simmer until the stock mixture is reduced by half (about 3–4 minutes).

In a small jar, mix a small amount of the evaporated milk with the cornflour to make a thin paste.

Stir the cornflour paste and the remaining evaporated milk into the reduced stock. Add the lemon zest, salt, pepper and parsley. Stir until thickened and smooth. The sauce should be the consistency of a thin custard.

In a hot frying pan, fry the marinara mix in the olive oil until just cooked through (3–4 minutes). Once cooked, spoon the marinara into the sauce and gently combine. Then add the hot drained pasta and toss to coat.

Serve hot, sprinkled with the parsley and dill.

Serving suggestion: Serve with a leafy green salad.

For a food nerd: Use wholemeal spaghetti.

1 Serve: 7.6g total fat • 1.8g saturated fat • 2318kJ (552 calories) • 64g carbohydrates • 55g protein • 2.4g fibre

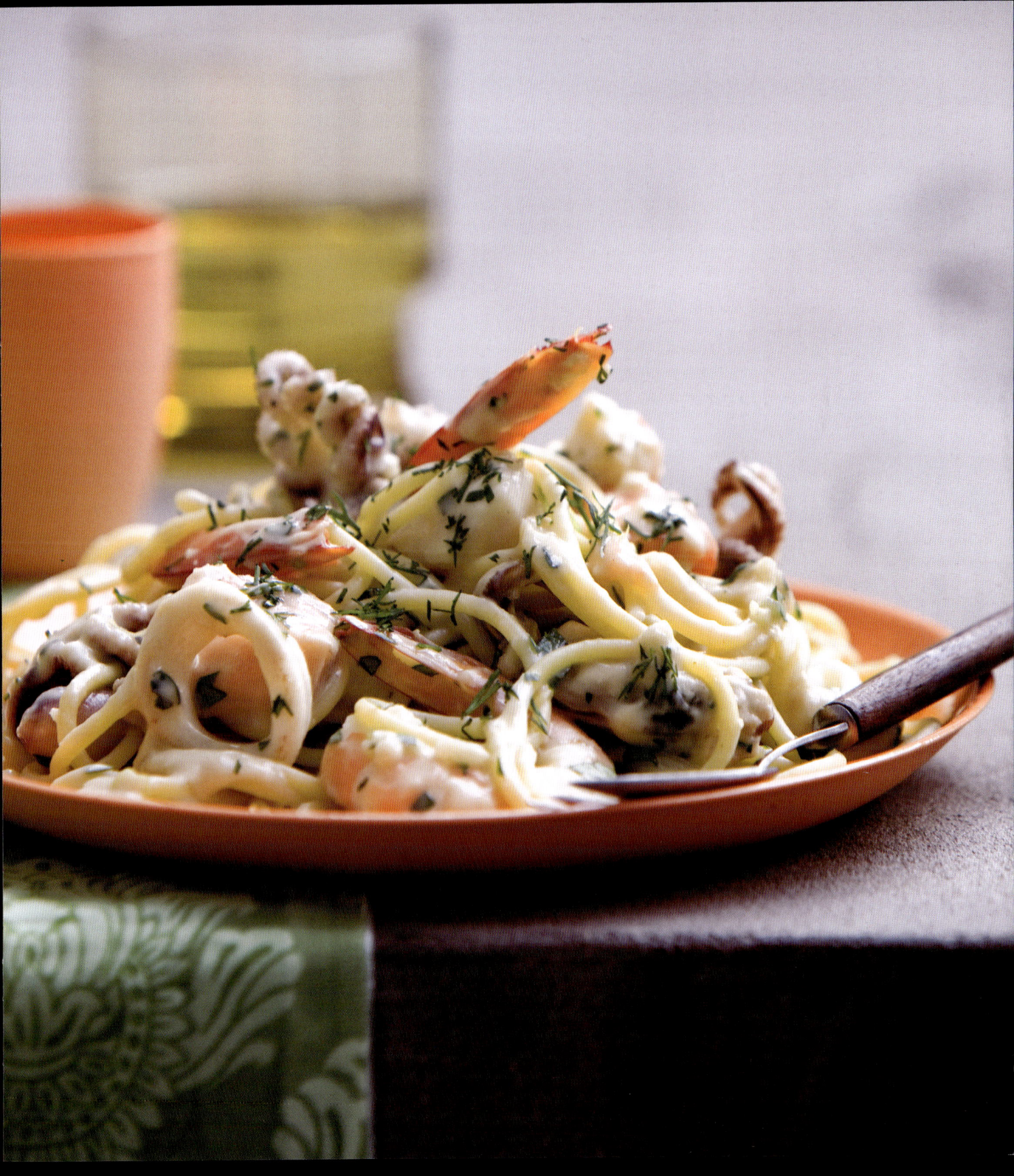

Cauliflower Cheese

Cauliflower, nutritionally a powerhouse, is closely related to broccoli and cabbage, all being part of the Brassicaceae vegetable family. The humble cauli is filled with the muscle building nutrient, potassium and is also rich in magnesium, phosphorous and manganese.

Serves: 4 • **Difficulty:** easy • **Takes:** 10 minutes to prep and 15 minutes to cook

4 large cauliflower florets
1 tablespoon shaved parmesan
 cheese

White Sauce
3 teaspoons cornflour
⅓ cup (80ml) skim milk, hot
1⅓ cup (330ml) boiling water
3 tablespoons grated low-fat
 cheddar cheese

Lemon Breadcrumbs
olive oil cooking spray
2 slices day-old wholemeal bread
1 garlic clove, crushed
2 teaspoons lemon zest

Set the oven at 180°C.

First make the breadcrumbs. Line a baking tray with baking paper and spray with the oil. Cut the bread into 1cm cubes and spread on the tray. Place in the oven for 10–15 minutes or until crunchy. Allow to cool, then crush roughly (leave some large pieces for texture, crunch and interest). Add the garlic clove and lemon zest. Set aside.

Steam the cauliflower until just tender (about 5 minutes). Place in a 15cm ovenproof dish and set aside.

To make the white sauce, combine the cornflour with 3 teaspoons of the hot milk. Then slowly add the rest of the hot milk and boiling water and stir. Place in a small saucepan over medium heat and gently cook, stirring constantly as the sauce thickens. Add the grated cheese and stir to combine.

Pour the sauce over the cauliflower. Crumble ¼ cup of the lemon breadcrumbs over the sauce and scatter the shaved parmesan on top.

Put the dish in the oven for 5–7 minutes, or until the cheese begins to melt.

Serving suggestion: Serve with grilled chicken breast or steak and steamed vegetables.

For a food nerd: Add broccoli and a ½ teaspoon of mustard to fire the flavour up.

1 Serve: 2.7g total fat • 1.5g saturated fat • 462kJ (110 calories) • 7g carbohydrates • 10g protein • 2.5g fibre

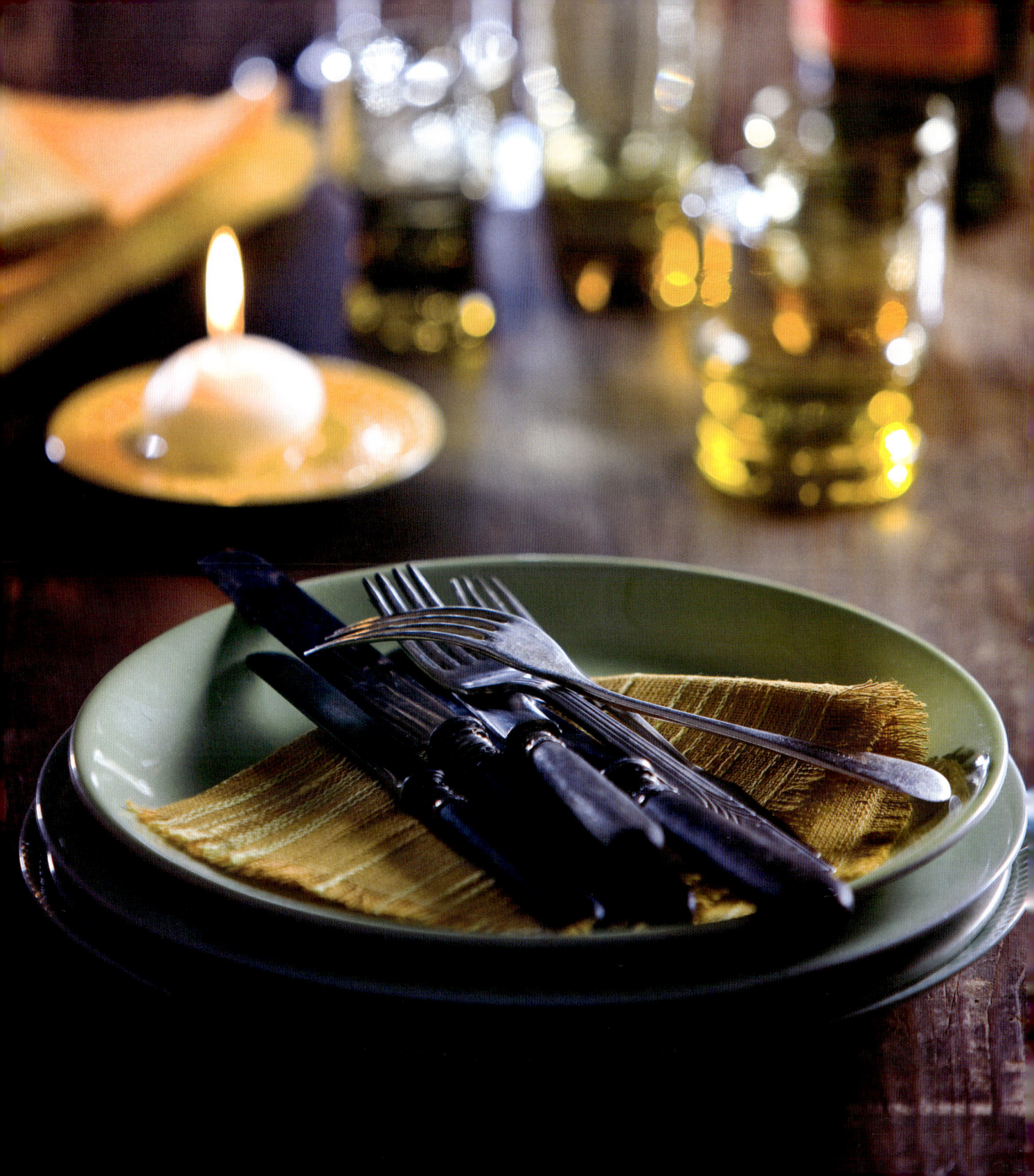

Bangers and Mash

Sausages can be a nutritional minefield, filled with fat, cheap meat, preservatives and additives. This is an extreme sausage makeover as you are making them from scratch, but they are quick and easy, and look even better if you have a sausage-making machine or a sausage-making attachment for your food processor.

Serves: 4 • **Makes:** 12 small sausages • **Difficulty:** easy • **Takes:** 15 minutes to prep, 10 minutes to cook

Sausages

400g extra lean organic minced beef

1 small onion, finely chopped

½ cup (60g) finely grated sweet potato

½ cup (50g) breadcrumbs

2 tablespoons barbecue sauce

1 teaspoon chopped oregano (or ½ teaspoon dried)

1 teaspoon chopped thyme (or ½ teaspoon dried)

½ tablespoon finely chopped flat-leaf parsley

Mash

2 large potatoes, peeled and roughly chopped

1 teaspoon good quality spread

1 tablespoon low-fat milk or evaporated skim milk

Set the oven at 180°C.

Combine all the sausage ingredients in a food processor and pulse until just combined. Don't over mix as it will make the mixture pasty.

Wet hands and roll approximately 1 tablespoon of mixture into a sausage shape. Repeat with the remaining mixture until finished.

Place the sausages on a baking tray lined with baking paper. Bake in the oven for 25–30 minutes until cooked through, turning halfway through.

Meanwhile, to make the mash steam the potatoes until just tender. Remove from the heat and drain well. Allow to cool slightly with the lid off. Place the potatoes over a low heat, add the spread and milk and mash to the desired consistency. Turn off heat and place the lid on potatoes until ready to serve.

Serving suggestion: Serve with rainbow salad (page 166) or Chinese greens with bean sprouts and mirin (page 162).

For a food nerd: Use orange mash (page 179) in place of the potato mash or use half potato and half white beans mashed together.

1 Serve: 18g total fat • 7g saturated fat • 1810kJ (431 calories) • 40g carbohydrates • 23g protein • 1g fibre

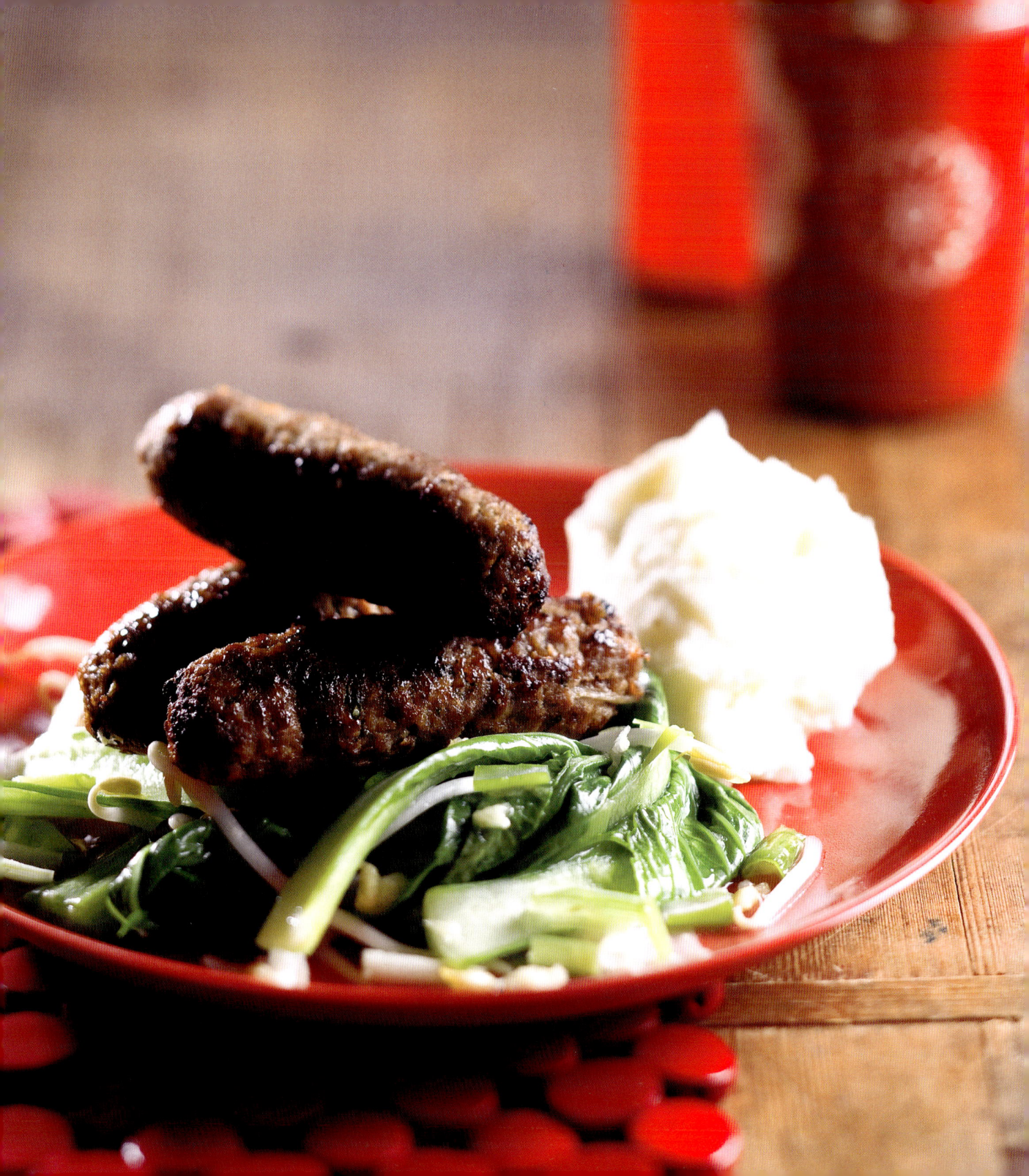

Cheesy Spinach Stuffed Pasta

There is something warm and homely about baked pasta dishes. They are also great to prepare ahead and heat up when you walk in the door late and need a quick, nutritious dinner. This dish tastes creamy and cheesy but evades the fat label because there is minimal oil used and all the cheeses are low-fat versions of the naturally low-fat white, fresh cheeses.

Serves: 4 • **Difficulty:** medium • **Takes:** 20 minutes to prep, 1 hour to cook

250g large pasta shells

Tomato Sauce
1 brown onion, diced

1 teaspoon extra virgin olive oil

1 clove garlic, crushed

2 x 400g tins diced tomatoes

2 tablespoons low-salt tomato paste

½ cup (125ml) low-salt vegetable stock

pinch of salt

1 teaspoon sugar

Filling
1 large bunch English spinach, washed, stalks removed, leaves roughly chopped (about 100g leaves)

2 spring onions, finely chopped

Set the oven at 180°C.

Cook the pasta shells in a large pan of boiling water for 3–4 minutes. Rinse and drain. The pasta will be softened but not cooked at this stage.

Steam the spinach until just beginning to wilt. Drain and set aside.

Make the tomato sauce by frying the onion with the olive oil in a frying pan for 2–3 minutes, or until the onion is soft. Add the garlic and cook while stirring for a further 2 minutes. Stir in the diced tomatoes, tomato paste, stock, salt and sugar. Bring to the boil, then simmer, covered, for 8–10 minutes.

Meanwhile, place all the filling ingredients in a bowl and mix thoroughly.

Spread the tomato sauce over the base of a 2-litre (8-cup) ovenproof dish. Add a small amount of extra stock if required to thin the sauce so it spreads easily.

Stuff each pasta shell with the spinach and cheese filling and pack the shells into the ovenproof dish so that they support each other and stand upright.

Cover with foil and bake for 1 hour, or until the pasta is tender and the tomato sauce is bubbling.

2 teaspoons finely chopped
  mint
2 tablespoons finely chopped
  flat-leaf parsley
¼ teaspoon ground nutmeg
2 eggs, lightly beaten
1 tablespoon tamari sauce
100g low-fat ricotta cheese
100g low-fat cottage cheese

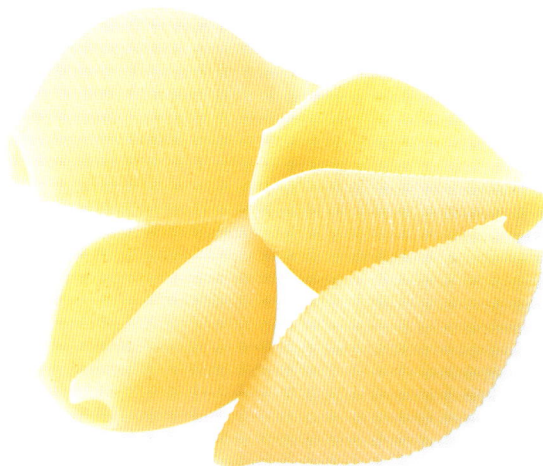

Serving suggestion: Serve with a green salad.

1 **Serve:** 7g total fat • 2.5g saturated fat • 1621kJ (386 calories) • 60g carbohydrates • 21g protein • 5.6g fibre

Lasagne

Where do you start when you do a lasagne makeover? The cheesy béchamel sauce, the lack of vegetables, the fatty mince meat, the extra cheese on top or the 33 grams of fat in every serve are all great places to begin. This lasagne recipe is delicious and the amount of béchamel sauce has been reduced to only using it on top of the dish, not on every layer, and by using a low-saturated-fat spread instead of butter and omitting the cheese from the sauce.

Serves: 6 • **Difficulty:** easy • **Takes:** 20 minutes to prep, 45 minutes to cook

400g lasagne sheets
¾ cup grated low-fat
   mozzarella cheese

Bolognese Sauce

2 teaspoons extra virgin
   olive oil
300g extra lean organic
   minced beef or chicken
½ cup grated pumpkin
½ cup grated sweet
   potato
1 carrot, grated
2 x 400g tins diced
   tomatoes
1 tablespoon low-salt
   tomato paste
2 teaspoons finely
   chopped oregano
2 teaspoons finely
   chopped thyme

To make the bolognese sauce, heat the olive oil in a large frying pan or electric saucepan to medium-hot. Add the meat and stir until browned, then add the pumpkin, sweet potato, carrot, tomatoes, tomato paste, oregano, thyme, paprika, salt and sugar. Bring to the boil, reduce heat to low and simmer for 20 minutes, covered, stirring occasionally. Stir in the parsley and basil, and simmer for a further 5 minutes.

To make the béchamel sauce, melt the spread in a medium sized saucepan. Once bubbling, add the flour, stirring constantly, and cook for 1 minute. Remove from heat and gradually add the stock and milk, constantly stirring to avoid it going lumpy. If lumps appear, whisk the mixture until smooth. Return to heat and stir until the sauce thickens.

Set the oven at 180°C.

To assemble the lasagne, cover the base of a lasagne dish with a thin layer of the bolognese sauce. Cover the bolognese sauce with a layer of pasta. Repeat, making three layers until all of the bolognese sauce is finished. Finish with a layer of pasta, then pour the béchamel sauce over the top and spread evenly to cover the pasta. Sprinkle the grated mozzarella over the top. Bake for 45–50 minutes, or until the cheese is melted and golden brown.

1 teaspoon paprika

pinch of salt

½ teaspoon sugar

1 tablespoon finely chopped
flat-leaf parsley

1 tablespoon finely chopped
basil

Béchamel Sauce

1 tablespoon good quality
spread

1 tablespoon wholemeal
plain flour

½ cup (125ml) low-salt
vegetable stock

½ cup (125ml) skim milk

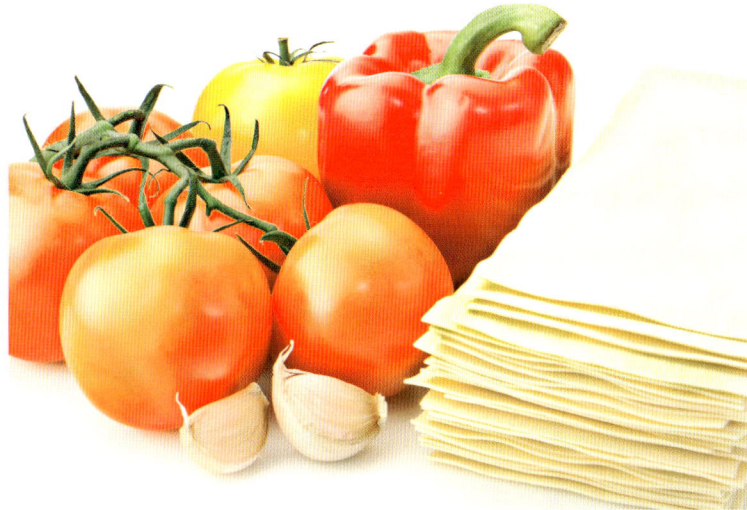

Serving suggestion: Serve with a rainbow salad (page 166).

For a food nerd: Add a cup of grated pumpkin, carrot and sweet potato and a cup of washed, drained and mashed tinned brown lentils to the bolognese sauce while it simmers. Reduce the minced meat to 250 grams.

1 Serve: 13g total fat • 4.8g saturated fat • 2041kJ (486 calories) • 67g carbohydrates • 24.5g protein • 4g fibre

Rich Scalloped Potatoes

Eggs, full-cream milk, cheese and full-fat cream are the four traditional ingredients in scalloped potatoes that pack it with nearly 30 grams of fat per serve. They taste delicious but are filled with saturated fat, kilojoules and not much else. Using egg whites, evaporated milk and low-fat cheese still gives you the same impressive golden bubbling dish and delicious taste but not the bad fats.

Serves: 10 • **Difficulty:** easy • **Takes:** 15 minutes to prep, 45 minutes to cook

500g potatoes, peeled and thinly sliced

1 clove garlic

1 cup (250ml) low-fat evaporated milk

2 egg whites, lightly beaten

½ teaspoon freshly grated nutmeg

pinch of salt

¼ teaspoon white pepper

½ cup (75g) grated low-fat mozzarella cheese

Set the oven at 180°C.

Rub a 33cm x 26cm ovenproof dish (like a lasagne dish) with the cut garlic. Arrange the potato slices in layers in the dish.

Mix the evaporated milk, egg whites, nutmeg, salt and pepper together, then pour over the potatoes. Sprinkle the grated cheese over the top and bake for 45 minutes, or until the potatoes are tender and golden.

Serving suggestion: Serve with a spicy dish, such as Thai fish cakes (page 121), and a salad of mixed green leaves.

For a food nerd: Use a mixture of potato, sweet potato and pumpkin to give this dish more colour, vitamins and minerals.

1 Serve: 1.1g total fat • 0.7g saturated fat • 619.5kJ (147.5 calories) • 29g carbohydrates • 6.7g protein • 3.3g fibre

Curried Sausages

Most sausages are cheap meat loaded with saturated animal fat. These days, there is much more selection and, if you shop carefully and choose well, you can buy sausages that contain good quality meat, are much lower in fat and salt than the traditional sausage and are still filled with flavour. Organic sausages are not much more expensive than good quality sausages but have the added benefit of not having any of the cheap, unwanted or artificial fillers that many conventional sausages can have.

Serves: 4 • **Difficulty:** easy • **Takes:** 15 minutes to prep, 1 hour to cook

6 organic extra lean beef
  sausages
1 teaspoon peanut oil
1 brown onion, sliced
2 tablespoons curry
  powder
1 cup (250ml) vegetable
  stock
400g tin diced tomatoes
4 celery stalks, chopped
2 carrots, cut into
  matchsticks
1 cup (155g) frozen peas

Place the sausages in a saucepan, cover with cold water and bring to the boil over high heat for 2 minutes. Simmer, then drain the sausages and allow them to cool slightly. Chop each sausage into five pieces.

Heat the oil in a large heavy-based saucepan over medium-hot heat. Add the onion and lightly fry until the onion is translucent and soft. Stir in the curry powder and fry for 1–2 minutes to release the fragrance. Add the sausage pieces and coat them with the onion and curry mix. Fry for 2–3 minutes.

Add the stock, tomatoes, celery and carrots and simmer for 5 minutes. Mix in the peas and cook for a further 7 minutes, uncovered, until the sauce thickens.

Serving suggestion: Serve with orange mash (page 179) or steamed brown rice and a rainbow salad (page 166).

For a food nerd: Only use four sausages and double the quantity of vegetables.

1 Serve: 7.6g total fat • 2g saturated fat • 680kJ (162 calories) • 16g carbohydrates • 8g protein • 4g fibre

Fettuccine Carbonara

It is the combination of fatty bacon, egg yolks, cream and high-fat cheese that puts fettuccine carbonara right near the top of the fat list with a huge 45 grams of fat per serve (25 grams of which are the artery clogging saturated fats). The traditional version has little going for it other than taste! Using 97% fat-free bacon, only one egg, low-fat evaporated milk and a small amount of the very flavoursome parmesan cheese gives this version fantastic taste *and* nutrition credentials.

Serves: 4 • **Difficulty:** medium • **Takes:** 5 minutes to prep, 15 minutes to cook

375g fettuccine

1 egg

375ml tin low-fat evaporated milk

olive oil cooking spray

2 garlic cloves, thinly sliced

4 rashers 97 per cent fat-free bacon, thinly sliced

2 tablespoons chopped chives

finely grated parmesan cheese

Cook the fettuccine in a large saucepan of boiling water for 12 minutes, or until *al dente*.

Meanwhile, whisk together the egg and evaporated milk. Set aside.

Spray a frying pan with the oil and heat over medium heat. Fry the garlic and bacon until soft. Remove from the pan and drain on absorbent paper.

Place the drained bacon and garlic back into the pan and, while off the heat, add the egg mixture, whisking quickly and constantly. Move the pan on and off the heat, while whisking, to ensure the egg cooks but does not scramble.

Once thickened, quickly add the chives and the pasta, and mix through.

Serve immediately with a small amount of grated parmesan cheese on top.

Serving suggestion: It is important to serve with a rainbow salad (page 166), mixed green leaves or another vegetable-rich side as there are no vegetables in this dish. The vegetables will help make it a complete meal, reduce your serve of carbonara and cut the richness of the dairy.

For a food nerd: Use wholemeal pasta for increased fibre.

1 Serve: 8g total fat • 3.3g saturated fat • 2016kJ (480 calories) • 81g carbohydrates • 25g protein • 3.3g fibre

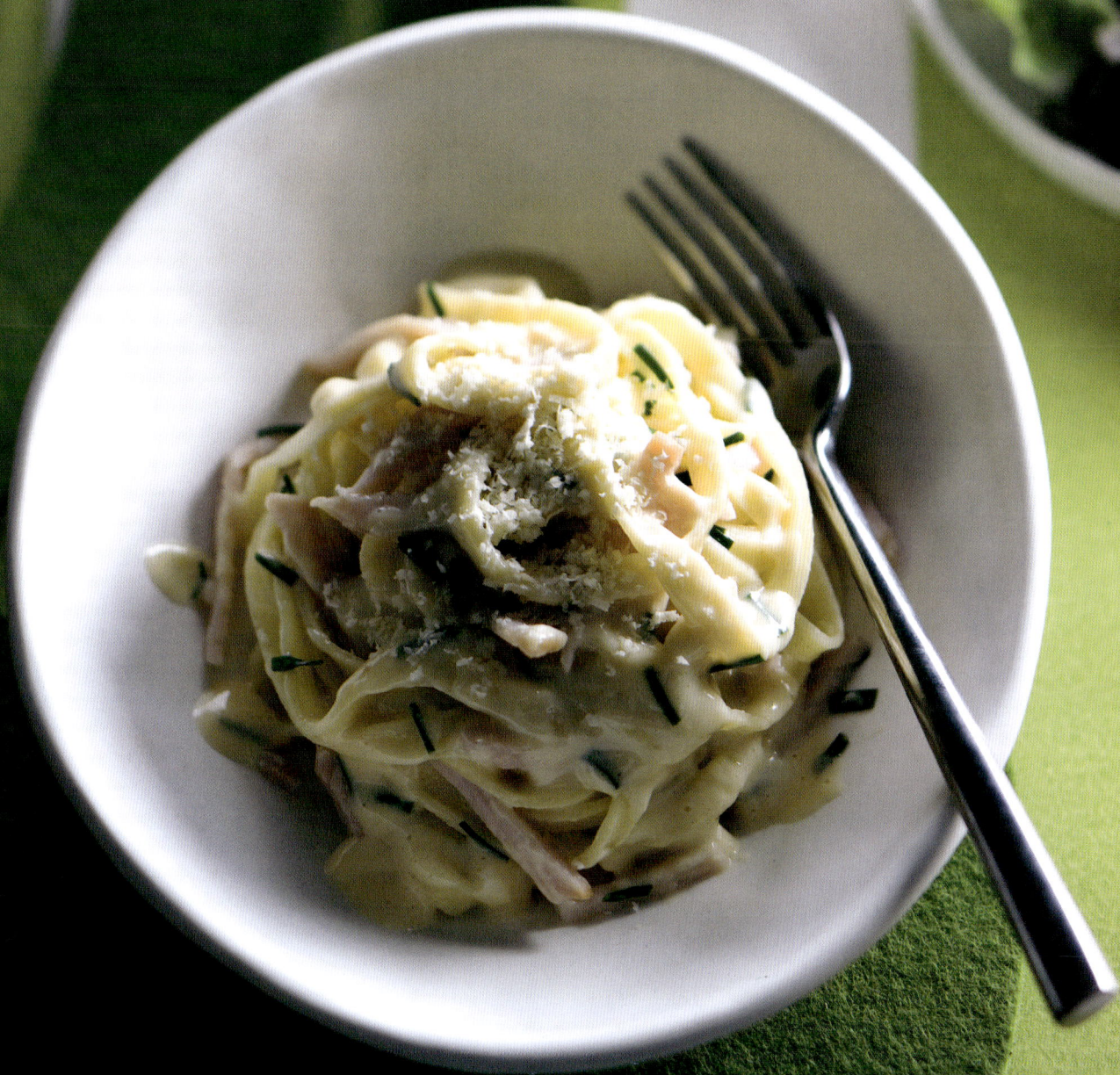

Cannelloni

These pasta tubes are usually stuffed with cheese, then sit in an oily tomato sauce hidden under another dose of more cheese. Reducing the amount of cheese, using low-fat varieties and cutting the oil in the tomato sauce does not diminish the flavour or the enjoyment of this dish at all. When you do remove or significantly reduce some central ingredients in a recipe, it is a good idea to focus on the herbs and spices you use and ensure they are working hard for you to cover any flavour gaps you may have created with your alterations. You will see many herbs working hard in the recipe below.

Serves: 6 • **Difficulty:** easy • **Takes:** 30 minutes to prep, 30–40 minutes to cook

200g packet cannelloni tubes

¼ cup (35g) low-fat mozzarella cheese, grated

Filling

1 teaspoon extra virgin olive oil

1 onion, finely diced

2 cloves garlic, crushed

500g extra lean organic minced beef

2 tablespoons low-salt tomato paste

½ teaspoon dried oregano

½ teaspoon dried thyme

1 bunch English spinach, washed, stalks removed, leaves roughly chopped

Set the oven at 180°C.

Make the filling first. Heat the oil in a large frying pan over medium-high heat. Fry the onion and garlic until the onion is soft. Add the meat and stir until browned. Mix in the tomato paste, oregano, thyme and spinach. Cook for 10 minutes, stirring occasionally.

In a jug, combine the egg white, evaporated milk, salt and pepper.

Pour the milk mixture into the pan and add the basil. Stir well to coat the meat and spinach. Cook for a further 2–3 minutes.

To make the tomato sauce, heat the oil in a frying pan over medium-hot heat. Fry the onion and garlic until the onion is soft. Add the tomatoes, tomato paste, salt and sugar. Bring to the boil, then reduce heat to low and simmer, covered, for 15 minutes.

1 egg white
¼ cup (60ml) low-fat
    evaporated milk
pinch of salt
4 grinds of black pepper
6 basil leaves, finely sliced

Tomato Sauce

1 teaspoon extra virgin
    olive oil
1 brown onion, diced
1 clove garlic, crushed
2 x 400g tins diced
    tomatoes
3 tablespoons low-salt
    tomato paste
pinch of salt
1 teaspoon sugar

To assemble, spread 4 tablespoons of the tomato sauce over the base of a 2-litre (8-cup) ovenproof dish. Pipe or stuff the cannelloni tubes with the filling and arrange them in a single layer on top of the tomato sauce in the dish. Continue layering until all the filled tubes are used, then spoon all the remaining tomato sauce over the cannelloni. Sprinkle the mozzarella cheese over the top and bake in the oven for 30–40 minutes, or until the cannelloni tubes are soft and the cheese is golden and melted.

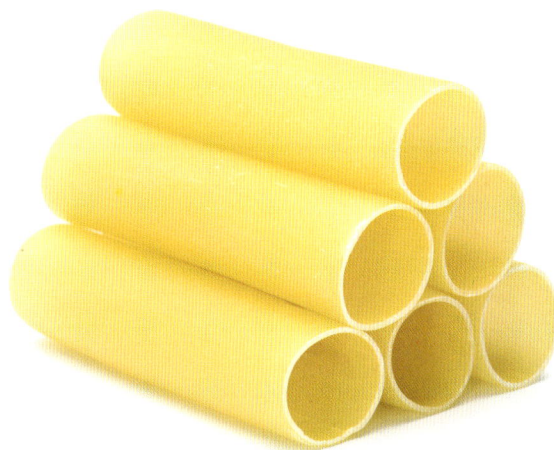

Serving suggestion: Serve with a green salad or a rainbow salad (page 166). This is also nice with a simple bowl of dressed iceberg lettuce.

1 Serve: 17g total fat • 6g saturated fat • 1168kJ (278 calories) • 11g carbohydrates • 20g protein • 1.5g fibre

Shepherd's Pie

Shepherd's pie is a hearty dish that traditionally uses lamb and has over 20 grams of saturated fat per serve. By using lean minced chicken and no cream or butter in the mash topping, it becomes a healthy dish that feeds the whole family on a budget.

Serves: 4 • **Difficulty:** easy • **Takes:** 20 minutes to prep, 45 minutes to cook

3 desiree potatoes, peeled and roughly chopped

½ cup (125ml) low-fat evaporated milk

freshly ground pepper

pinch of salt

¼ teaspoon nutmeg

1 teaspoon extra virgin olive oil

1 onion, diced

2 cloves garlic, crushed

500g extra-lean organic minced chicken, beef or lamb

2 teaspoons Worcestershire sauce

2 tablespoons barbecue sauce

1 teaspoon finely chopped oregano

1 teaspoon finely chopped thyme

1 teaspoon finely chopped flat-leaf parsley

⅔ cup (160ml) vegetable stock

Set the oven at 180°C.

Steam the potatoes until tender. Drain, then return the potatoes to the saucepan and cook, stirring, for 2 minutes until dry.

In a small saucepan, gently heat the milk. Do not boil. Pour the warmed milk onto the potatoes and mash until smooth. Add the pepper, salt and nutmeg. Set aside.

Heat the oil in a hot frying pan over medium heat and fry the onion and garlic until soft. Stir in the mince and fry until browned. Add the Worcestershire sauce, barbecue sauce and herbs. Then pour in the vegetable stock and simmer for 5 minutes or until the sauce is slightly thickened.

Spoon the meat sauce into a 1-litre (4-cup) ovenproof dish. Completely cover with the mashed potato, and, using a spoon, make peaks on the potato. Bake for 45 minutes until golden on top.

Serving suggestion: Serve with tamari cauliflower and broccoli (page 175) or Chinese greens with bean sprouts and mirin (page 162).

For a food nerd: Use sweet potato instead of potato for the mash. Sweet potato is lower on the glycemic index and is a great source of vitamins A and C, iron, calcium and fibre.

---

1 Serve: 6.9g total fat • 1.8g saturated fat • 1386kJ (330 calories) • 36g carbohydrates • 31g protein • 4.2g fibre

Hearty Beef Stew

It is the fatty meat and the added fat that makes beef stew stodgy and unhealthy, so using lean meat and getting your flavour from herbs and spices and not from added fat is the best way to give a hearty stew a makeover.

Serves: 4 • **Difficulty:** easy • **Takes:** 15 minutes to prep, 1 hour to cook

500g lean organic beef steak, trimmed of fat and diced into chunks

¼ cup (30g) plain flour

1 teaspoon extra virgin olive oil

1 brown onion, diced

3 cloves garlic, crushed

4 celery stalks, cut into 2cm pieces

3 carrots, diced

1 large potato, cut into chunks

1 teaspoon dried thyme

1 teaspoon dried oregano

1 bay leaf

1 tablespoon Worcestershire sauce

½ teaspoon freshly ground black pepper

400g tin diced tomatoes

1 cup (250ml) low-salt beef stock

Toss the meat in the flour to coat.

Heat the olive oil in heavy-based saucepan over medium-high heat. Add the meat and brown. Stir in the onion, garlic, celery, carrots and potatoes.

Add the herbs, Worcestershire sauce, pepper, tomatoes and stock and cook on low heat for up to 1 hour, or until the meat is tender.

If the stew appears to be sticking to the pan, add ½ cup (125ml) of water.

Remove the bay leaf and serve hot.

Serving suggestion: Serve with orange mash (page 179).

For a food nerd: Add an extra 1½ cups of vegetables to the stew and reduce the beef to 300g.

1 Serve: 11.5g total fat • 4.1g saturated fat • 1483kJ (353 calories) • 19g carbohydrates • 41.5g protein • 3g fibre

Beef Stroganoff

Beef stroganoff is rich and creamy, true comfort food for many. By heavily cutting the amount of sour cream used and only using extra-light sour cream, you still get the creaminess but not the fat. The leanness of the meat also helps to halve the fat of the traditional recipe and make this recipe fab.

Serves: 4 • **Difficulty:** medium • **Takes:** 15 minutes to prep, 15 minutes to cook

1 teaspoon extra virgin olive oil

500g organic rump steak, fat removed and cut across the grain into thin strips

1 medium brown onion, cut into thin wedges

3 garlic cloves, crushed

300g button mushrooms, cleaned and sliced (about 12 mushrooms)

2½ teaspoons cornflour

150g extra-light sour cream

2½ tablespoons tomato paste

¾ cup (185ml) low-salt vegetable stock

2 tablespoons finely chopped flat-leaf parsley

Heat the oil in a large, heavy-based frying pan over medium-high heat. Stir-fry the meat in two batches for 2 minutes or until just cooked. Remove from the pan. Set aside.

Reduce heat to medium and fry the onion and garlic for 3–4 minutes or until soft. Add the mushrooms and cook for a further 3–4 minutes, or until soft.

Combine the cornflour, sour cream and tomato paste in a jug. Add the stock and combine.

Pour the sauce into the frying pan and stir well. Simmer for 5 minutes, stirring occasionally, to allow the sauce to thicken.

Return the meat to the pan and stir well. Cook for a couple of minutes until the meat is warmed through.

Sprinkle the parsley on top and serve.

Serving suggestion: Serve with steamed brown rice or orange mash (page 179).

For a food nerd: Serve with tamari cauliflower and broccoli (page 175) or rainbow salad (page 166) to boost the vegetable content of the meal.

1 **Serve:** 13g total fat • 4.8g saturated fat • 1453kJ (346 calories) • 14g carbohydrates • 44g protein • 2g fibre

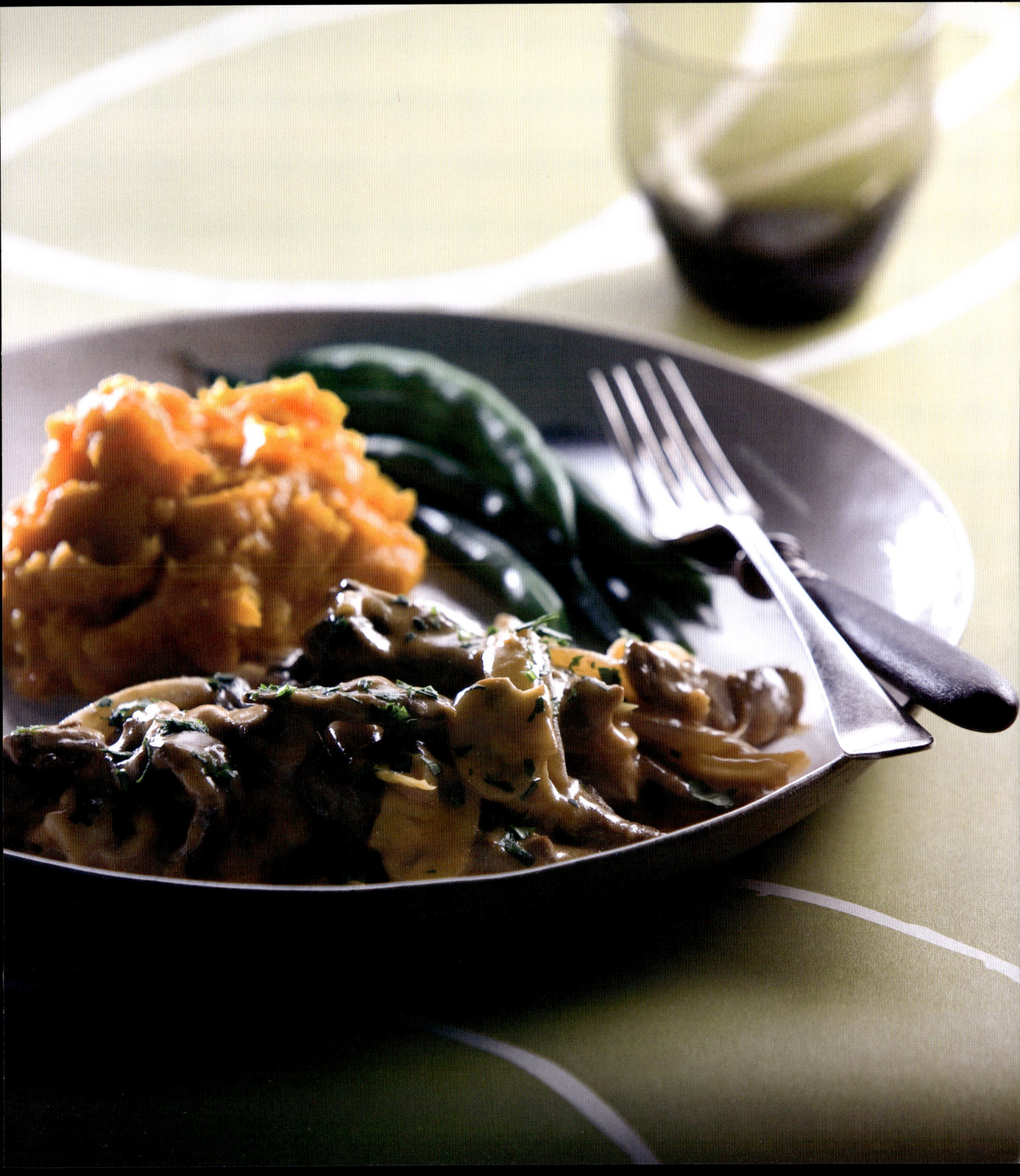

Fab eating out

Fab eating needs to work in your everyday life and most of us love to eat out, so here is a guide to eating out while staying on the straight and narrow.

Portion size, salt, fat, sugar and kilojoules are the usual suspects when you eat out.

Top tips

- Don't clear your plate if you are given a large meal. Stop when you are full (and give your stomach time to tell you that you are full).

- Talk to the waiter if you are unclear about the ingredients or the cooking methods.

- Order your salads with the dressing on the side so you can easily control how much dressing you use.

- If you are really hungry, opt for a healthy starter so you can skip dessert.

- If you choose to have dessert, wait until you finish your main meal before you order it.

- Maximise your vegetables by ordering a side salad with no dressing or choosing a wrap instead of a big roll, focaccia or Turkish bread.

- Don't over order. Ask the waiting staff how big the serves are and order more when, and if, you need it.

- When buying work lunches, try baked potato, tomato-based pasta, or wraps. Watch out for cheesy and creamy dressings and sauces, pastry, deep-fried foods and mayonnaises. Many places now stock low-fat or low-salt versions of sauces and condiments, just ask. Decline the upsize, even if it is only one dollar more. Resist the temptation to have chips and a soft drink on the side of your healthy order as they will undo all your good work.

There is a lot of grey area between the 'Avoid' list and the 'Try' list but the following table will guide you in making sensible decisions.

Avoid	Try
Deep-fried, battered, sautéed, au gratin, buttery, creamy, hollandaise, alfredo, parmesan, gravy, hash, pot pie, crispy, cheesy	Grilled, boiled, poached, steamed, stir-fried, broiled, baked, garden fresh
Fatty meats and antipasti, like salami, bacon, sausages	Lean meat such as chicken and kangaroo; fish, seafood, steak; and pulses like beans
Pastry such as pies, quiches, croissants, cakes, biscuits,	Bread, especially wholemeal, wholegrain or high fibre
Cream and cheese-based sauces	Tomato-based sauces
Curries, such as green curries, based on coconut milk	Curries with no coconut milk
Dressed salads and vegetables	Salads and vegetables with dressings on the side
Fried rice	Steamed or boiled rice
Creamy desserts, puddings, cakes, sweet pastries and rolls	Fruit-based desserts such as fruit salad, sorbet, gelato or a fruit plate

The best and the worst of it

Thai
The best
Stir-fried vegetable dishes with some added chicken, fish or seafood; stir-fried noodles; lean Thai salads, for example beef salad or spicy squid salad; steamed rice; stock-based soups, such as hot and sour prawn soup, without coconut milk.

The worst
Deep-fried starters such as salt and pepper squid, fish cakes, curry puffs; red and green curries based on coconut milk; curries that include peanuts.

Italian
The best
Pizza topped with vegetables and half the regular amount of cheese; bread sides such as bruschetta and grissini; tomato-based pasta sauces such as bolognese or arrabiata accompanied by a side salad without dressing; fruit-based starters such as prosciutto and melon; non-creamy soups such as minestrone; fruit-based desserts such as sorbet or gelato.

The worst
Deep-fried meat (chicken and veal are commonly deep-fried in Italian cuisine), dishes with a high butter or oil content such as garlic bread or antipasto; dishes containing large amounts of cheese or creamy sauces such as cannelloni and lasagne; cream-based sauces such as carbonara, alfredo and some marinara sauces; dishes containing fatty meats such as sausage, bacon and meat-lovers pizza; pizzas made with lots of cheese such as stuffed-crust pizzas or three-cheese pizzas.

Japanese

The best
Fresh fish and vegetable dishes such as noodle soups, sukiyaki, sashimi and sushi (California rolls, maki rolls, inari; onigiri); traditional sides such as miso soup, edamame, chawanmushi and seaweed salad; fresh salads with no dressing; lean meat dishes such as yakitori, teriyaki beef or teriyaki chicken.

The worst
Deep-fried dishes such as tempura or chicken or pork katsu.

Indian

The best
Dishes, like tikka or tandoori, that use herbs and spices rather than creamy sauces for flavour. Dishes based on vegetables and legumes such as dhal; low-fat sides such as steamed or pilau rice, naan bread, chapatti, lime pickle, grilled pappadams or yoghurt raita. Request that no oil be added to the sides.

The worst
Creamy or very oily dishes such as butter chicken, chicken or vegetable biryani or korma, masala and pasanda curries; deep-fried sides such as pakoras, fried pappadams, meat samosas or onion bhajis.

Chinese

The best
Vegetable or lean meat based stir-fries such as black bean, oyster sauce, chop suey, chow mein (ask for rice instead of the fried noodles) or Szechwan; steamed or poached dishes such as steamed chicken or seafood, dumplings and steamed dim sum or rice; stock- or water-based soups such as chicken or crab and sweetcorn soup and wonton noodle soups.

The worst
Deep-fried dishes and sides such as sesame prawn toast, battered sweet and sour pork, prawn crackers, fried dim sum, spring rolls, fried rice, crispy duck pancakes, anything with battered or crispy in the dish name.

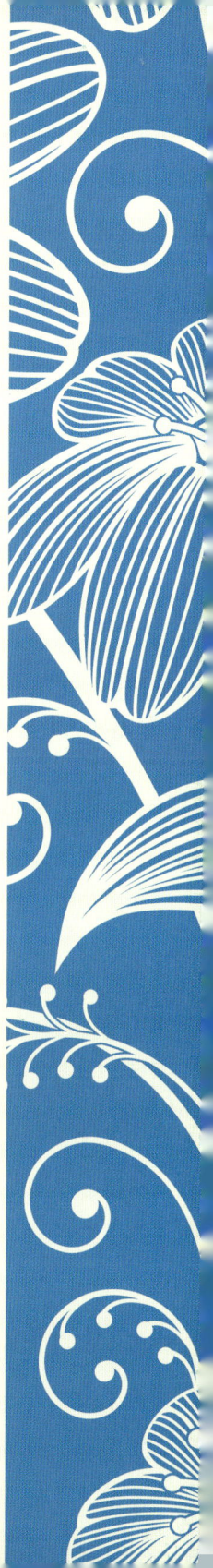

Fried Rice

By reducing the oil, boosting the vegetables, using lean, good quality meat and brown rice you can make fried rice a great dinner option. The key to making this recipe a success is to cook the rice the day before and keep it in the fridge until you need it. Cook your brown rice until it is tender and no longer chewy. This takes between 30–40 minutes. If you cook it well, you will notice very little difference between using white and brown rice, but the brown rice will really boost the dish's fibre.

Serves: 4 • **Difficulty:** easy • **Takes:** 30 minutes to prep, 30 minutes to cook

2 eggs, beaten

¼ cup (60ml) chicken stock

2 tablespoons tamari or low-salt soy sauce

1 teaspoon grated fresh ginger

2 teaspoons extra virgin olive oil

6 spring onions, finely chopped

1 clove garlic, crushed

3 rashers 97% fat-free bacon

3 celery stalks, diced

3 carrots, diced

½ red capsicum, diced

1 fresh corn cob, slice the kernels off

5 cups (925g) day-old cooked rice (this is 2 cups uncooked)

1 cup (155g) frozen peas

Combine the eggs, stock, tamari or soy and ginger in a jug.

Heat the oil in a wok over medium-high heat and add the spring onions, garlic and bacon. Stir-fry for 3–4 minutes. Add the celery, carrots, capsicum and corn and stir-fry for a further 5 minutes until the celery and carrots are just tender. Add the rice and peas, toss to mix well.

While constantly tossing the rice mixture, gradually add the chicken-stock mixture, and cook for a further 5 minutes, or until the rice is completely heated through and the eggs are cooked.

For a food nerd: If you are looking to limit your carbohydrates, reduce the amount of rice and boost the vegetables. Add dried shiitake mushrooms for a good winter immunity boost. Soak them for 30 minutes in a small bowl of warm water, then squeeze out the excess water and slice the mushrooms before you throw them into the rice.

---

1 Serve: 10g total fat • 3g saturated fat • 1877kJ (447 calories) • 74g carbohydrates • 16.6g protein • 9g fibre

Spring Rolls

The filling in spring rolls varies from mysterious pork pieces to just cabbage. They do have one thing in common, they are all deep-fried and filled with grease. Surprisingly, they work very well in the oven and so don't have the fat from the fryer, making them a great weekend night treat.

Serves: 7 • **Makes**: 14 spring rolls • **Difficulty**: easy • **Takes**: 30 minutes to prep, 15 minutes to cook

14 frozen spring roll
   wrappers, thawed
olive oil cooking spray

Filling

2 teaspoons vegetable oil
300g skinless chicken
   breast fillets, diced
2 cloves garlic, crushed
½ cup (40g) finely
   shredded Chinese
   cabbage
1 small carrot, finely
   grated
1 teaspoon grated ginger
2 tablespoons hoisin
   sauce

Set the oven at 220°C.

To make the filling, heat the oil in a frying pan over medium-high heat and add the chicken and garlic. Stir-fry until the chicken is nearly cooked. Add the cabbage, carrot, ginger and hoisin sauce. Cook for 3–4 minutes, or until the cabbage is limp and the carrot is just tender. Allow to cool.

Place a tablespoon of the cooled filling in one corner of a wrapper and roll three times to enclose the filling. Cut the remaining wrapper off then brush the edges of the spring roll with water to ensure the wrapper stays closed. Repeat until all the rolls are made.

Spray a lined baking tray with the oil and place the spring rolls on the tray in a single layer. Spray the rolls with more oil.

Place in the oven for 5–7 minutes, then turn the rolls and bake for another 5–7 minutes.

Serving suggestion: Serve with some steamed brown rice and stir-fried greens.

For a food nerd: Use low-salt tamari, not soy sauce, as a dipping sauce.

1 Serve: 2g total fat • 0.4g saturated fat • 504kJ (120 calories) • 12g carbohydrates • 12g protein • 0.6g fibre

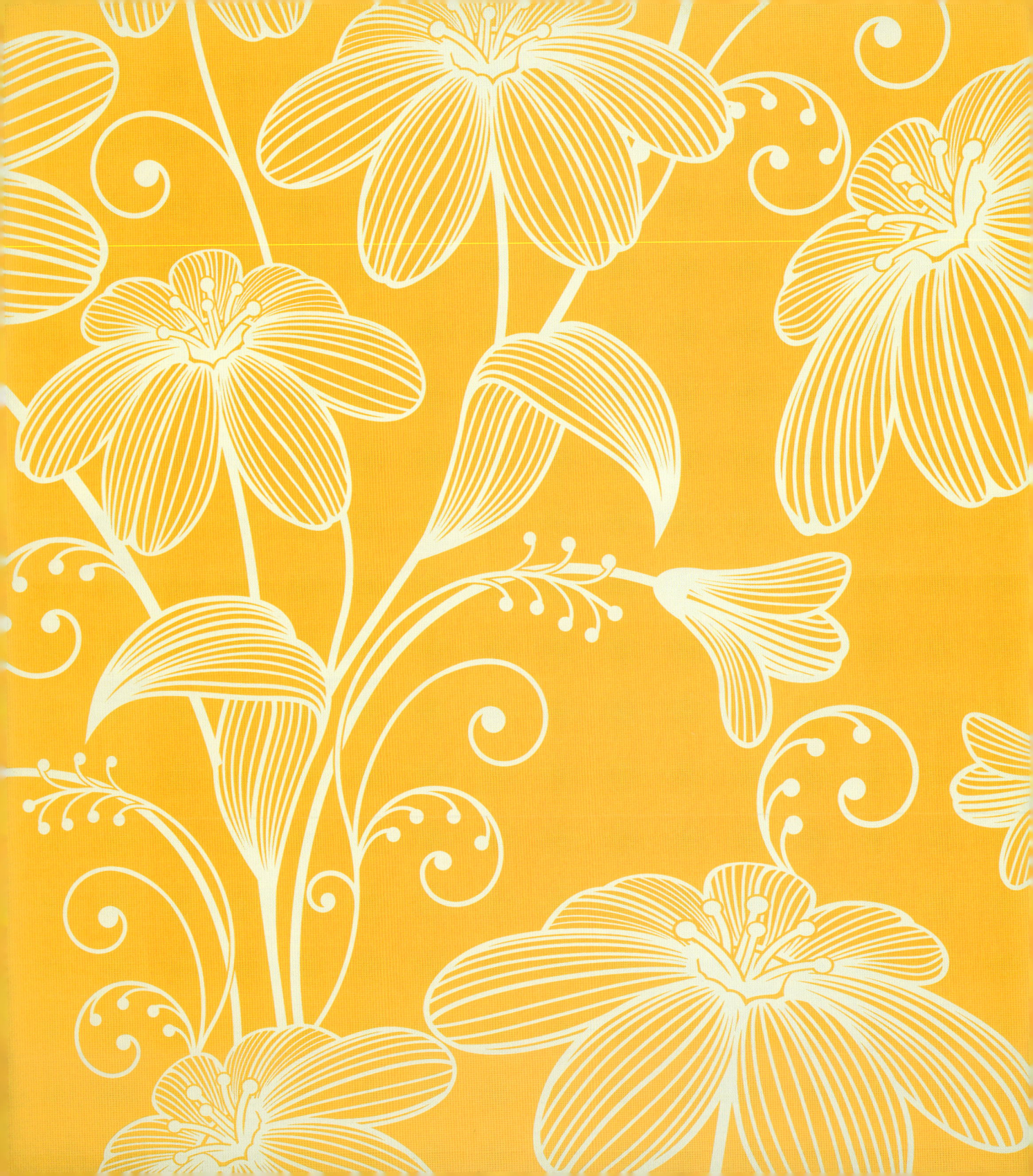

Five-Star Sides

Even the fab versions of some meals are not a fantastic complete-meal option. To turn them into a complete meal, serve them up with one or two of these five-star sides, so you can enjoy your favourites guilt free. These sides are all nutritional pocket rockets, so that even your pasta carbonara, when served with a five-star side or two, will give your body a real hit of the good stuff.

They are written to be easy, quick and appeal to even the most vegetable phobic. You will not even know you are eating veggies, they are so tasty. They are a great way to get people not used to eating veggies, eating them by giving them variety. If you are already a big vegetable eater (good on you), they will give you lots of ideas and inspiration to try new things. Most of them are coated with delicious, healthy dressings and sauces that are heart-friendly versions of the traditional fat dressings, and they are wonderful at disguising some of the veggie tastes you may not love.

The chapter starts with the salad sides for summer and spring and then follows with some warm sides to help you get through autumn and winter. Where oil is needed, I recommend extra virgin olive oil but you could use flaxseed (linseed) oil or a nut oil, as these are rich in nutrients.

The addition of one or two of these sides will always add an extra star to your meal's fab rating.

Rocket, Pear and Pea Salad

Leafy green vegetables are one of the very best foods you can regularly include in your diet. They are rich in numerous vitamins and minerals, and have fantastic plant compounds (phytochemicals) which help us ward off disease. Many people would rather feed them to rabbits but if you know how to use them and serve them with complementary flavours and a healthy dressing, then they are an easy and extremely healthy addition to your diet. Try this rocket, pear and pea salad, then rotate it with the other three options listed below. When you make the dressing, double the amount and keep it in a jar in the fridge for the next night and another greens option.

Serves: 4 • **Difficulty:** easy • **Takes:** 5 minutes to prep

1 large bunch rocket, washed and dried

1 ripe Williams or beurre bosc pear, cored, quartered and sliced lengthways

¾ cup (115g) frozen peas, thawed

Dressing

¼ cup (60ml) red or white balsamic vinegar

2 teaspoons extra virgin olive oil or nut oil

2 teaspoons wholegrain mustard

Combine the rocket, sliced pear and peas in a bowl.

Place the vinegar, oil and mustard in a glass jar, put the lid on and shake to combine well. Pour the dressing over the salad and toss through just before serving.

For a food nerd: Use the same dressing, but vary the salad ingredients depending on what is in season. Try watercress, flat-leaf parsley and grated raw beetroot; or endive, radicchio, spring onions and sliced green beans; or baby spinach, mint, green beans and peas.

1 Serve: 2.8g total fat • 0.4g saturated fat • 315kJ (75 calories) • 12g carbohydrates • 2g protein • 2.6g fibre

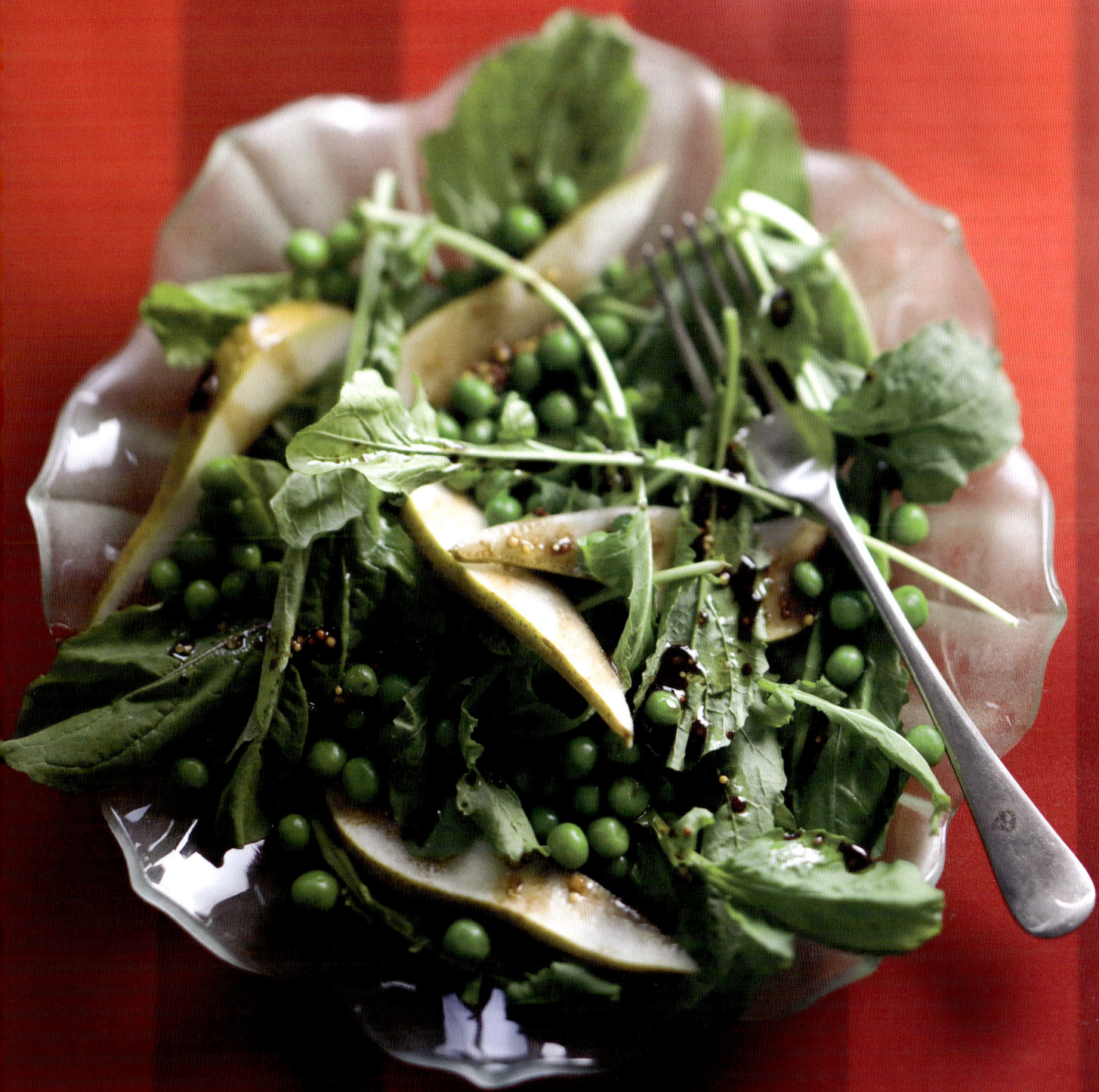

Coleslaw

For a great coleslaw, shred the cabbage very finely, mix well with the leek, red onion and carrot and dress it, then leave it for 10 minutes to allow the flavours to marry and develop.

Serves: 4–6 • **Difficulty:** easy • **Takes:** 10 minutes to prep

2 cups (150g) finely shredded white savoy or red cabbage

1 celery stalk, finely diced

1 large carrot, grated

¼ cup (35g) washed and finely diced leek

½ red apple, unpeeled

Dressing

2½ tablespoons low-fat natural yoghurt

1½ tablespoons good quality low-fat mayonnaise

¼ teaspoon paprika

1 teaspoon mustard powder or Dijon mustard

In a large bowl, combine the cabbage, celery, carrot and leek.

Place all the dressing ingredients in a small jar, put on the lid and shake to combine well.

Just before serving, cut the red apple into matchsticks and gently mix into the cabbage.

Place all the dressing ingredients in a jar and shake well.

Pour the dressing over the coleslaw and toss well to coat the ingredients.

Serve immediately.

For a food nerd: Add 1½ tablespoons of freshly chopped flat-leaf parsley to boost the iron.

1 Serve: 0.4g total fat • 0.1g saturated fat • 168kJ (40 calories) • 8g carbohydrates • 2g protein • 2g fibre

Asparagus with Parmesan

Fresh asparagus in season is a very good accompaniment to a meal. It only needs to be lightly fried as it is nicest eaten warm but still crispy.

Serves: 4 • **Difficulty:** easy • **Takes:** 5 minutes to prep, 5 minutes to cook

2 bunches asparagus, washed and trimmed
1 teaspoon extra virgin olive oil
freshly ground black pepper
1 tablespoon finely grated parmesan cheese

Cut the asparagus in half.

Heat a medium sized frying pan over high heat and add the olive oil.

Toss the asparagus in the hot pan, add the pepper, and stir-fry for 3–4 minutes, or until it turns bright green but is still crisp.

Remove from the pan and sprinkle with the parmesan cheese.

Serve immediately.

1 Serve: 1.7g total fat • 0.4g saturated fat • 143kJ (34 calories) • 4g carbohydrates • 2g protein • 2g fibre

Chinese Greens with Bean Sprouts and Mirin

Chinese greens include bok choy, choy sum, wombok (Chinese cabbage) and any of those leafy greens you see in the Asian greens section in the fruit and vegetable shop. They are all suitable for this recipe. They are nutrition dynamos, but are not widely used in Australia as many people don't know how to make them tasty. Mirin is a sweet Japanese cooking wine. It is available from supermarkets and fruit and vegetable shops. You could also use Shaoxing, fermented Chinese rice wine, also available from supermarkets, or a small amount of dry sherry.

Serves: 4 • **Difficulty:** easy • **Takes:** 5 minutes to prep, 5 minutes to cook

olive oil cooking spray

2 spring onions, sliced lengthways and roughly chopped

2cm piece ginger, finely grated

2 garlic cloves, crushed

2 cups bean sprouts, washed

1 large bunch bok choy, choy sum or wombok, washed and roughly chopped

3 tablespoons mirin

Heat a large frying pan or wok sprayed with the oil over medium-high heat. Add the spring onions, ginger and garlic and stir-fry for 2 minutes, or until just beginning to soften. Don't allow the garlic to brown or it will become bitter.

Add the bean sprouts and Chinese greens and stir-fry until they begin to collapse but still maintain their bright green colour.

Pour in the mirin and stir-fry for another minute.

Serve warm.

For a food nerd: Add 1 cup of finely sliced broccoli.

1 **Serve:** 0.1g total fat • 0g saturated fat • 265kJ (63 calories) • 13g carbohydrates • 4.5g protein • 1g fibre

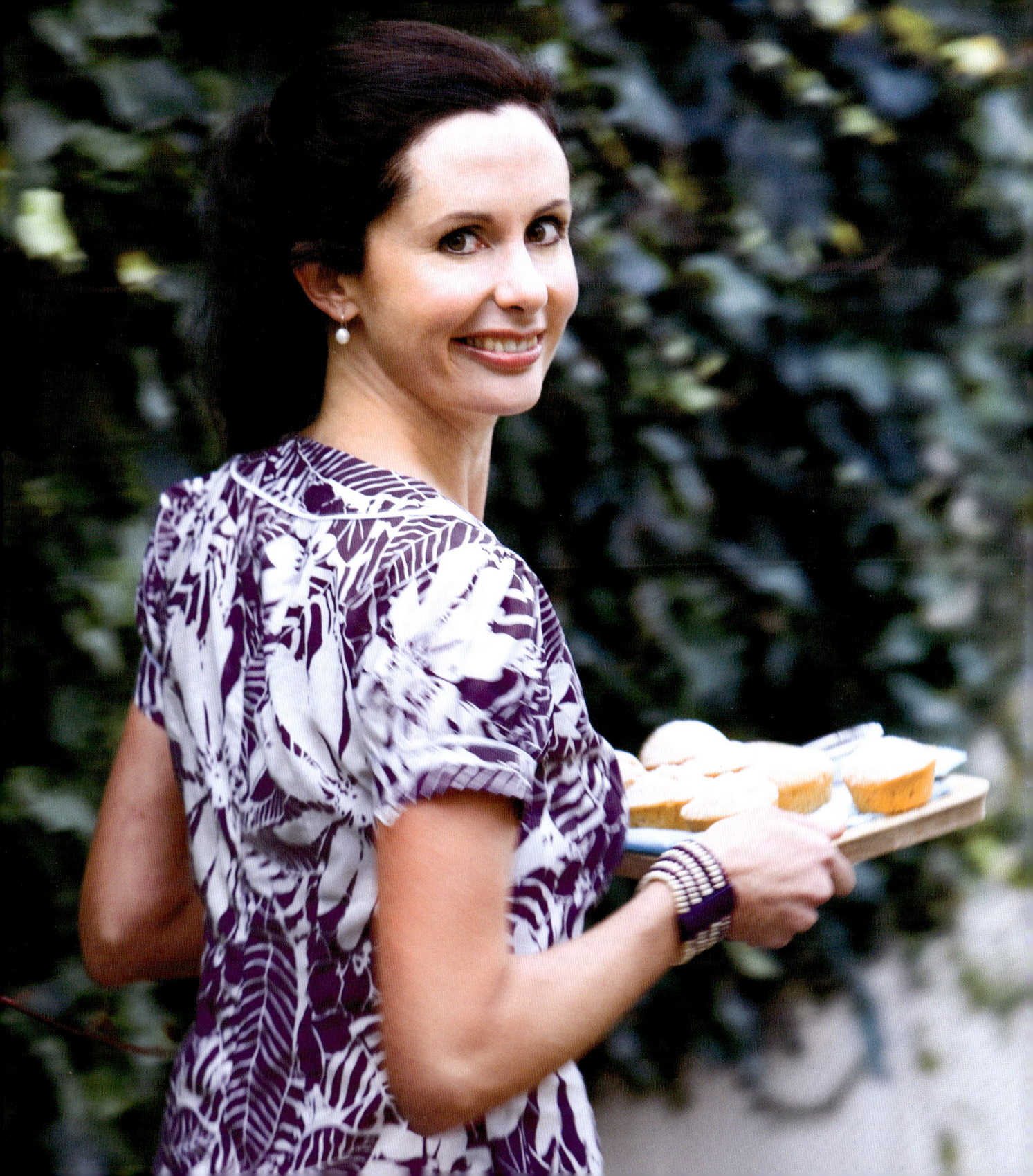

Red Salsa

This spicy salsa is quick to make and is a great accompaniment to meat dishes or it can be used as a dip for crackers.

Serves: 2 • **Difficulty:** easy • **Takes:** 5 minutes to prep, 20 minutes to stand

3 tomatoes, finely diced
1 tablespoon finely
   sliced red onion, or
   3 spring onions, finely
   sliced
1 teaspoon sweet chilli
   sauce

Mix all the ingredients together and place in the fridge for 20 minutes to allow the flavours to develop.

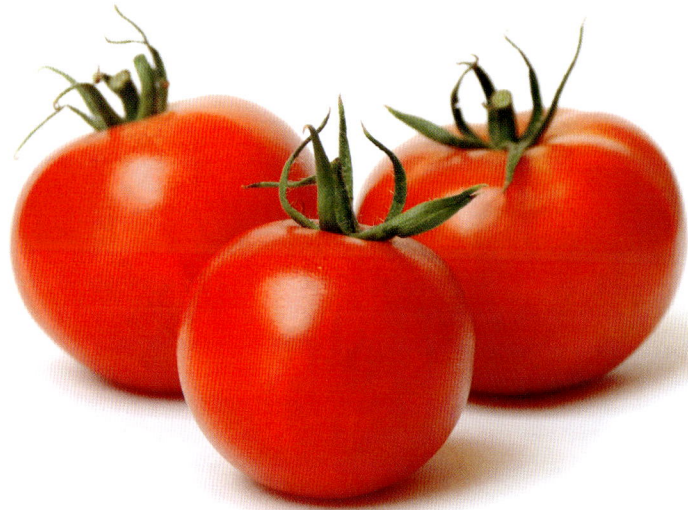

For a food nerd: Add 1 tablespoon of finely chopped red capsicum and ½ clove of garlic, crushed.

1 Serve: 0.6g total fat • 0.1g saturated fat • 199.5kJ (47.5 calories) • 10.6g carbohydrates • 2g protein • 2g fibre

Green Salsa

When making this salsa, keep the white membranes of the capsicum in the salsa. We often cut them out but they contain lots of nutrients. This salsa is very spicy, so cut down on the chilli if you want to keep it mild.

Serves: 4 • **Difficulty:** easy • **Takes:** 5 minutes to prep

2 Lebanese cucumbers, diced

½ cup (80g) finely diced green capsicum

1 green chilli, deseeded and finely chopped

2 tablespoons finely chopped flat-leaf or curly parsley

juice of lemon or lime

½ teaspoon ground cumin

2 spring onions, finely sliced

½ avocado, peeled and diced

Combine all the ingredients in a medium sized bowl. Serve.

Serving suggestions: Add low-fat cottage cheese or natural yoghurt and serve on crackers for lunch.

For a food nerd: Use the dark green part of the spring onions as well as the white for a boost of chlorophyll and other nutrients.

1 Serve: 3.6g total fat • 0g saturated fat • 291kJ (69.4 calories) • 9.5g carbohydrates • 2g protein • 3g fibre

Without the avocado: 0.3g total fat • 0g saturated fat • 139kJ (33 calories) • 7.7g carbohydrates • 1.5g protein • 1.5g fibre

Rainbow Salad

This is like a garden salad but using as many different salad vegetables as you have in the fridge. Using lots of different vegetables will give you a range of colours and so give you lots of different vitamin and mineral combinations. It also makes the salad taste different each time you make it. Some ideas for ingredients are listed below but your imagination is the limit for this one – the more variety the better.

Serves: as many people as you like • **Difficulty:** easy • **Takes:** 10 minutes to prep

cherry tomatoes
corn kernels fresh from the cob
carrot, grated
cucumber, sliced
raw beetroot, finely grated
mixed green leaves
iceberg lettuce
red or green capsicum, diced or
  sliced
peas, snow or snap or frozen
  garden peas
broccoli florets, blanched
green beans, finely sliced

Dressing
2 tablespoons apple juice
1 tablespoon white wine
  vinegar
1 teaspoon Dijon mustard

Make enough for each person to have 1 cup or 1½ cups if this is the only vegetable dish you are serving.

Combine the salad ingredients in a large bowl and toss well.

Place the dressing ingredients in a small glass jar, put on the lid and shake well.

Dress the salad and serve immediately.

Serving suggestions: For a complete meal, add a tin of washed and drained chickpeas, cannellini beans, or four bean-mix or some chopped boiled eggs.

Nutritional information per serving dependent on combination of ingredients used.

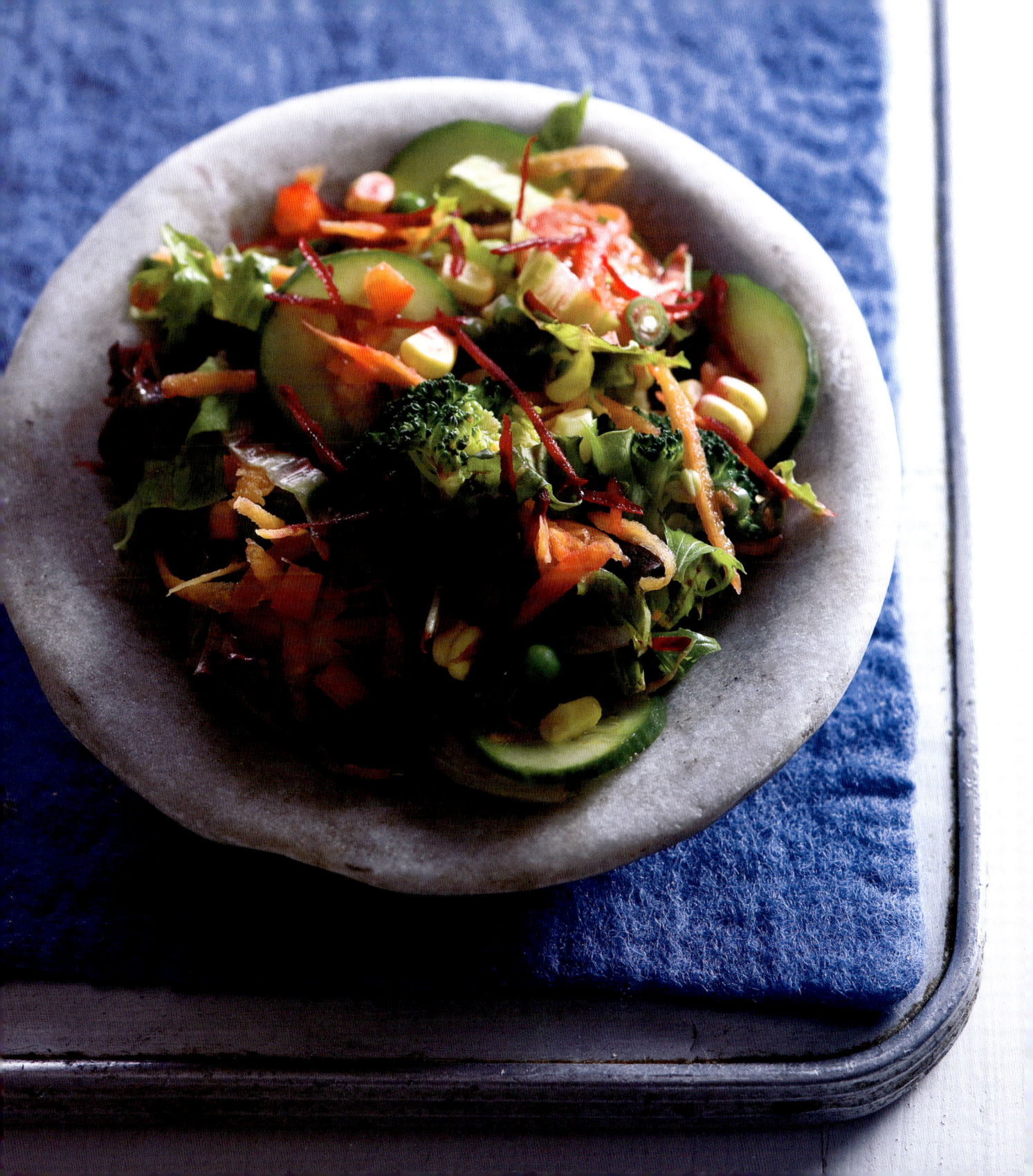

Moroccan Bean Salad

This is a fabulous way to serve legumes and thereby boost the nutrition (especially the fibre and protein) of any meal. The dressing is only mildly spicy but adds a real kick to the beans, and is a very easy way for someone not used to cooking with legumes to introduce them into their diet. Always use the whole spring onion as the dark green ends are filled with chlorophyll, a fantastic nutrient. If you add some baby spinach or other dark green salad leaves, this would make a great lunch.

Serves: 4–6 • **Difficulty:** easy • **Takes:** 10 minutes to prep, 10 minutes standing time

420g tin of four- or five-
   bean mix, rinsed and
   drained
2 spring onions, thinly sliced
¼ cup (80g) finely diced red
   or green capsicum
1 large tomato, diced
1 tablespoon finely chopped
   flat-leaf or curly parsley
1 teaspoon finely chopped
   mint

Dressing
½ clove garlic, crushed
½ teaspoon ground cumin
¼ teaspoon paprika
pinch of salt
pinch of cayenne pepper
1 tablespoon lemon juice
1 teaspoon extra virgin
   olive oil

In a medium sized bowl place the beans, spring onions, capsicum, tomato, parsley and mint. Gently mix together.

To make the dressing, place the garlic, cumin, paprika, salt, cayenne pepper, lemon juice and olive oil in a glass jar. Put the lid on and shake well.

Pour the dressing over the bean salad and stir through.

Leave to stand for 10 minutes before serving.

1 Serve: 1.4g total fat • 0.2g saturated fat • 433kJ (103 calories) • 14g carbohydrates • 6g protein • 6g fibre

Cucumber Raita

This is a fantastic accompaniment to any Indian dishes, curries or spicy meals.

Serves: 4 • **Difficulty:** easy • **Takes:** 5 minutes to prep

2 Lebanese cucumbers, diced

1 cup (250g) low-fat or no-fat Greek yoghurt

1 teaspoon ground cumin

1 teaspoon ground mustard seeds

½ teaspoon paprika

1 tablespoon finely chopped mint

Combine all the ingredients in a bowl.

Serve with hot curries and spicy foods.

For a food nerd: Add 2 tablespoons of chopped flat-leaf or curly parsley to boost the iron.

1 Serve: 0.2g total fat • 0.1g saturated fat • 122kJ (29 calories) • 5g carbohydrates • 2.6g protein • 1.2g fibre

Caprese Salad

This is a wonderful way to serve tomatoes throughout the summer. Traditionally, a caprese salad has a slice of fresh mozzarella or bocconcini on top of each tomato slice. The cheese has been omitted from this recipe to keep the fat down. The fresh basil and tomatoes pack enough of a flavour punch without the cheese.

Tomatoes are full of lycopene, a known anti-cancer fighter. This salad tastes best with freshly picked basil leaves, so plant a bunch in a sunny spot in the back garden or get a pot going on your balcony.

Serves: 4 • **Difficulty:** easy • **Takes:** Less than 5 minutes to prep

4 ripe tomatoes, thickly
   sliced
1 bunch fresh basil,
   washed and leaves
   picked
1½ tablespoons balsamic
   vinegar
1 teaspoon extra virgin
   olive oil
freshly ground black
   pepper

Place the tomato slices on a plate.
   Place a fresh basil leaf on top of each tomato slice.
   Drizzle with the balsamic vinegar and oil.
   Sprinkle with black pepper to taste and serve.

1 **Serve:** 1.7g total fat • 0.2g saturated fat • 210kJ (50 calories) • 2g carbohydrates • 1.6g protein • 2g fibre

Potato Salad

Who doesn't love potato salad? The great news is that cold potato is filled with resistant starch (the third type of fibre) and so it will not load you up with carbohydrates. It is an excellent way to have potato without the carb side effects, but still keep an eye on your portion size.

Serves: 4–6 • **Difficulty:** easy • **Takes:** 5 minutes to prep, 10 minutes to cook, plus fridge cooling time

3 large waxy potatoes
1 tablespoon finely
   sliced spring onions
   (optional)

Dressing

2½ tablespoons low-fat
   natural yoghurt
1 tablespoon low-fat
   good quality
   mayonnaise
1 tablespoon finely
   shredded basil leaves
1 tablespoon lemon juice
1 teaspoon lemon zest

Steam the potatoes until just tender (around 10–12 minutes), drain and allow them to cool.

Make the dressing by placing all the ingredients in a small glass jar. Put the lid on and shake well. Pour the dressing over the cooled potatoes and gently coat. Sprinkle with the spring onions.

Cover and refrigerate until cold.

1 Serve: 0.3g total fat • 0.1g saturated fat • 651kJ (155 calories) • 34g carbohydrates • 5g protein • 4g fibre
This nutritional panel would alter considerably if the potatoes were chilled before serving. The calories and carbohydrate levels would reduce and the fibre would increase.

Harissa Rice Salad

Harissa-style dressings are hot and spicy — the perfect way to bring a rice salad alive. If you are not a fan of spicy food, then use the coleslaw dressing (page 160) or the rainbow salad dressing (page 166).

Remember to serve the salad cold, so that the rice is a source of resistant starch (fibre), not carbohydrates.

Serves: 6 • **Difficulty:** easy • **Takes:** 10 minutes to prep, plus fridge cooling time

1 cup (210g) uncooked brown rice, or 2 cups (370g) cooked brown rice
2 spring onions, finely sliced
1 celery stalk, diced
½ cup (80g) finely diced red capsicum
8 cherry tomatoes, quartered
½ cup (70g) thinly sliced fennel
½ cup torn basil leaves

Dressing

¼ teaspoon cayenne pepper
½ tablespoon ground cumin
½ teaspoon paprika
1 tablespoons tomato paste
2 tablespoons lemon juice
1 clove garlic, crushed
1 tablespoon extra virgin olive oil or flaxseed oil

Cook the rice until tender (around 30–40 minutes). Rinse, drain and allow to cool.

In a large bowl, combine the cooled rice, spring onions, celery, capsicum, cherry tomatoes, fennel and basil.

To make the dressing, place all the ingredients into a large glass jar, put on the lid and shake until well combined.

Pour the dressing over the salad and refrigerate.

Serve cold.

1 Serve: 3g total fat • 0.4g saturated fat • 508kJ (121 calories) • 22g carbohydrates • 2.6g protein • 2.5g fibre
This nutritional panel would alter considerably if the rice was chilled before serving. The calories and carbohydrate levels would reduce and the fibre would increase.

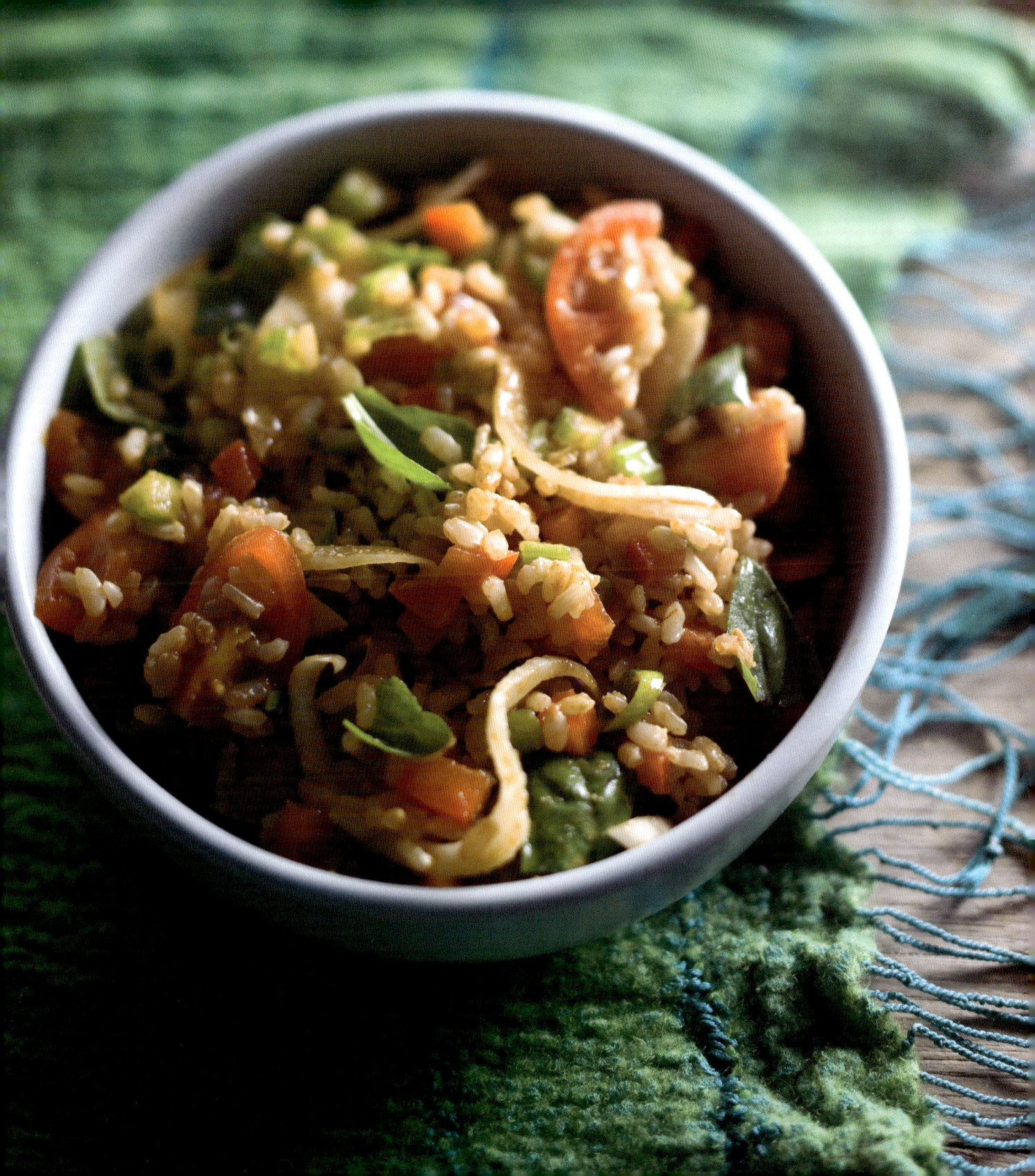

Pasta Salad

Like the potato salad and the rice salad, this one needs to be served cold to be a great source of resistant starch fibre. It can be served as a side dish or packed up in a lunchbox.

Serves: 6 • **Difficulty:** easy • **Takes:** 10 minutes to prep, plus fridge cooling time

250g wholemeal spiral pasta

410g can unsweetened corn
   kernels, drained

½ small red onion, finely diced

1 cup (155g) frozen peas,
   thawed

2 celery stalks, finely diced

½ cup (80g) finely diced
   green capsicum

100g green beans, finely
   chopped (about 24 beans)

2 tablespoons finely chopped
   flat-leaf parsley

Dressing

1 tablespoon good quality
   low-fat mayonnaise

2 tablespoons low-fat or
   no-fat Greek yoghurt

1½ teaspoons wholegrain
   mustard

1 teaspoon lemon zest

2 tablespoons buttermilk or
   skim milk

Cook the pasta until it is just *al dente*. Drain and allow to cool.

Place the pasta, corn, onion, peas, celery, capsicum, beans and parsley in a large bowl and mix.

Combine all the dressing ingredients in a small glass jar, put on the lid and shake well.

Pour the dressing over the salad ingredients and toss to combine.

Serve cold.

For a food nerd: Vary the grain of pasta you use each time you make this salad. Try buckwheat, corn, rice or spelt for different nutrients.

1 Serve: 1.4g total fat • 0.3g saturated fat • 659kJ (157 calories) • 33g carbohydrates • 8g protein • 6g fibre
This nutritional panel would alter considerably if the pasta was chilled before serving. The calories and carbohydrate levels would reduce and the fibre would increase.

Tamari Cauliflower and Broccoli

These two are the kings of vegetables, so any way you can boost them in your diet is fantastic. Even those who despise broccoli and cauliflower will love them done this way. Tamari is a natural, wheat-free soy sauce. It is still quite high in salt, so use it sparingly but you only need a small amount to give vegetables a real flavour hit. For a change, replace the tamari with one tablespoon of sweet chilli sauce.

Serves: 4 • **Difficulty:** easy • **Takes:** 5 minutes to prep, 5 minutes to cook

- 1 teaspoon extra virgin olive oil
- 4 cups broccoli florets
- 4 cups cauliflower florets
- 2 cloves garlic, crushed
- 1 tablespoon salt-reduced tamari or salt-reduced soy sauce

Heat a frying pan over high heat and add the olive oil. Toss the broccoli, cauliflower and garlic into the pan and stir-fry for 2–3 minutes. Add about ¼ cup of water and continue to cook for a further 2–3 minutes, or until just softening but still crunchy. Add the tamari or soy and toss for a further minute.

Serve hot.

For a food nerd: Add 1 cup of bean sprouts and some celery cut into julienne. Use the broccoli stalks as well as the heads as they are packed with vitamins and minerals.

1 Serve: 1.7g total fat • 0.2g saturated fat • 269kJ (64 calories) • 10.6g carbohydrates • 5g protein • 5g fibre

Roast Vegetables

Roast vegetables need to be crispy and lightly browned, but when they are roasted in the fat of the roasting meat, they are filled with saturated fat and any other nasties that drain out of the meat. To avoid this, spray them with some good quality olive oil and roast them on their own. This really cuts the fat down but still gives the crunchy, caramelised taste we all love. The rosemary gives them an added flavour dimension. Always use olive oil as it gives a much crunchier finish to the vegetables than other spray oils.

Serves: 4 • **Difficulty:** easy • **Takes:** 5 minutes to prep, 35-40 minutes to cook

500g pumpkin, peeled and
   cut into large chunks
1 large sweet potato, peeled
   and cut into large chunks
1 turnip or swede, peeled and
   cut into large chunks
2 red onions, halved
olive oil cooking spray
1½ tablespoons finely
   chopped rosemary

Set the oven at 200°C. Pat the chopped vegetables with a clean tea towel to ensure they are dry.

Line two baking trays with baking paper. Spray the paper with the oil and arrange the vegetables on the trays in a single layer. Spray the tops of the vegetables with the oil and sprinkle with the rosemary.

Bake for 15–20 minutes and then turn the vegetables so they brown on all sides. Cook for another 15–20 minutes, or until the vegetables are cooked through and golden.

For a food nerd: Toss the warm roasted vegetables into a bowl of rocket, mizuna or other dark green leaves and serve as a warm roasted salad. If you want to dress it, use the simple dressing on the rainbow salad (page 166).

1 Serve: 1.4g total fat • 0.2g saturated fat • 487kJ (116 calories) • 25g carbohydrates • 3g protein • 5g fibre

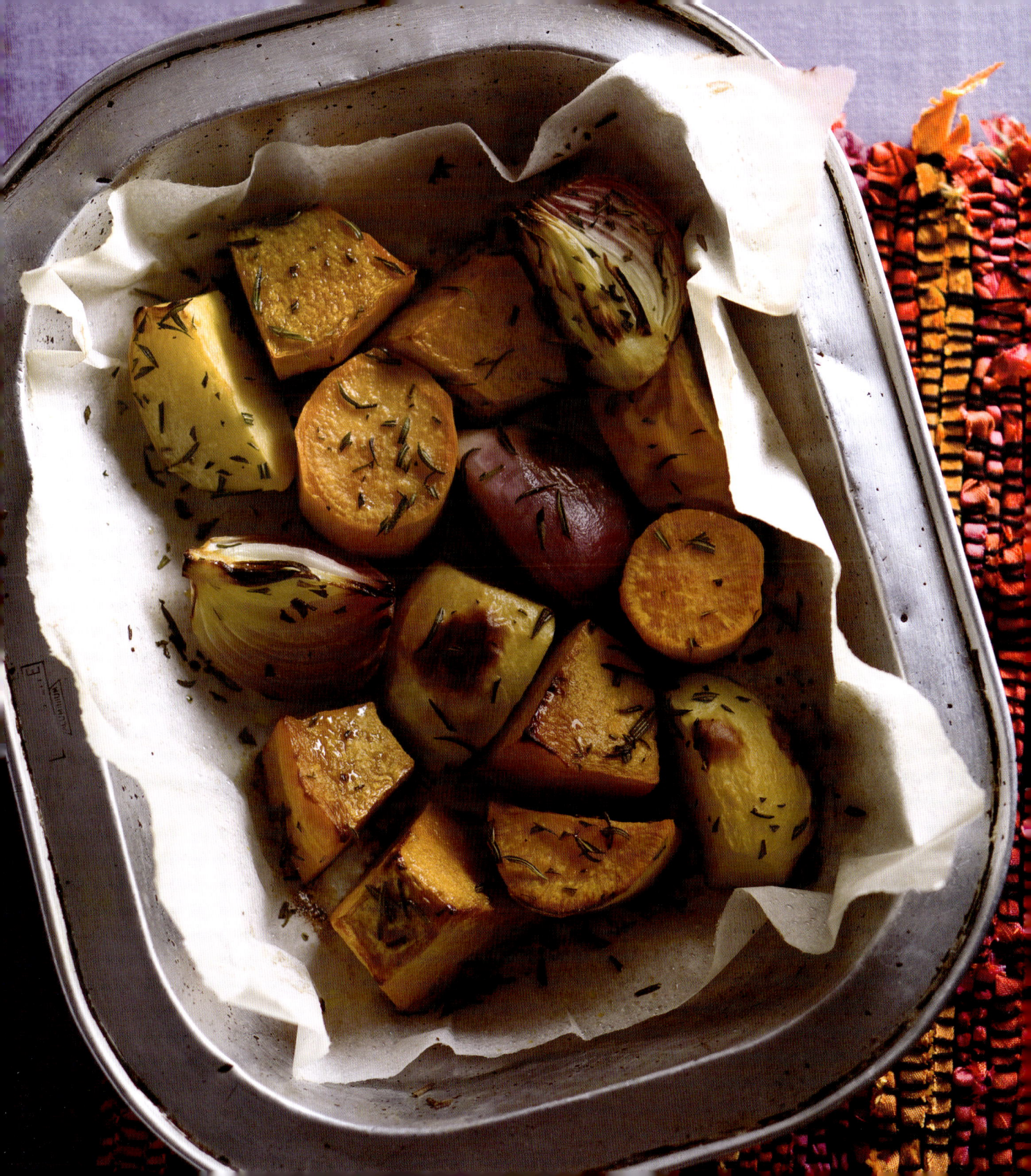

Ratatouille

This is a large recipe, but even if you are only cooking for one or two, cook the full amount and freeze it for an instant side filled with vegetables or an instant vegetable-filled pasta sauce. The longer you cook this ratatouille, the more the flavours deepen and develop.

Serves: 4-6 • **Difficulty:** easy • **Takes:** 10 minutes to prep, 25–30 minutes to cook

1 teaspoon extra virgin
   olive oil
1 small brown or red onion,
   finely sliced
2 cloves garlic, crushed
1 medium zucchini, chopped
   into 1cm rounds
1 Lebanese eggplant (smaller,
   longer variety) or half a
   larger eggplant, diced
400g tin diced tomatoes or
   10 fresh tomatoes, diced
2 tablespoons tomato paste
1 teaspoon oregano
   (or ½ teaspoon dried)
1 teaspoon thyme
   (or ½ teaspoon dried)
2 tomatoes, extra
pinch of salt
¼ teaspoon cayenne pepper
½ tablepoon red wine vinegar
1 teaspoon sugar
1 bay leaf

Heat the oil in a large frying pan over medium-high heat. Add the onion and garlic and lightly fry for 2–3 minutes, or until just soft.

Add the zucchini and eggplant and cook for a further 2–3 minutes. Then add the rest of the ingredients and simmer for a further 20 minutes on low, to allow the sauce to reduce and the flavours to develop. Stir occasionally.

Remove the bay leaf before serving.

For a food nerd: Add some kidney beans and serve this as a fresh, highly nutritious pasta sauce or jacket potato topping.

1 Serve: 1g total fat • 0.2g saturated fat • 256kJ (61 calories) • 12.5g carbohydrates • 2g protein • 3g fibre

Orange Mash

This is a great mash alternative to the high carbohydrate and high GI white potato mash. It is much richer in nutrients and is brimming with vitamin A and beta-carotene.

Serves: 4 • **Difficulty:** easy • **Takes:** 5 minutes to prep, 10 minutes to cook

4 carrots, peeled and
  chopped
300g pumpkins peeled
  and chopped
1 medium sweet potato,
  peeled and chopped
1 teaspoon good quality
  spread
pinch of nutmeg
  (optional)
freshly ground black
  pepper

Steam the vegetables until tender (8–10 minutes). Place them in a large bowl, add the spread, nutmeg and pepper, and mash until smooth.

  Serve hot.

1 Serve: 0.7g total fat • 0.2g saturated fat • 332kJ (79 calories) • 18g carbohydrates • 2g protein • 4g fibre

Compare this orange mash to ordinary mashed potato to see the big difference and this doesn't even show the huge boost of vitamin A and other nutrients you get from the orange mash.

Mashed potato: 0.7g total fat • 0.1g saturated fat • 911kJ (217calories) • 48g carbohydrates • 5.6g protein • 6g fibre

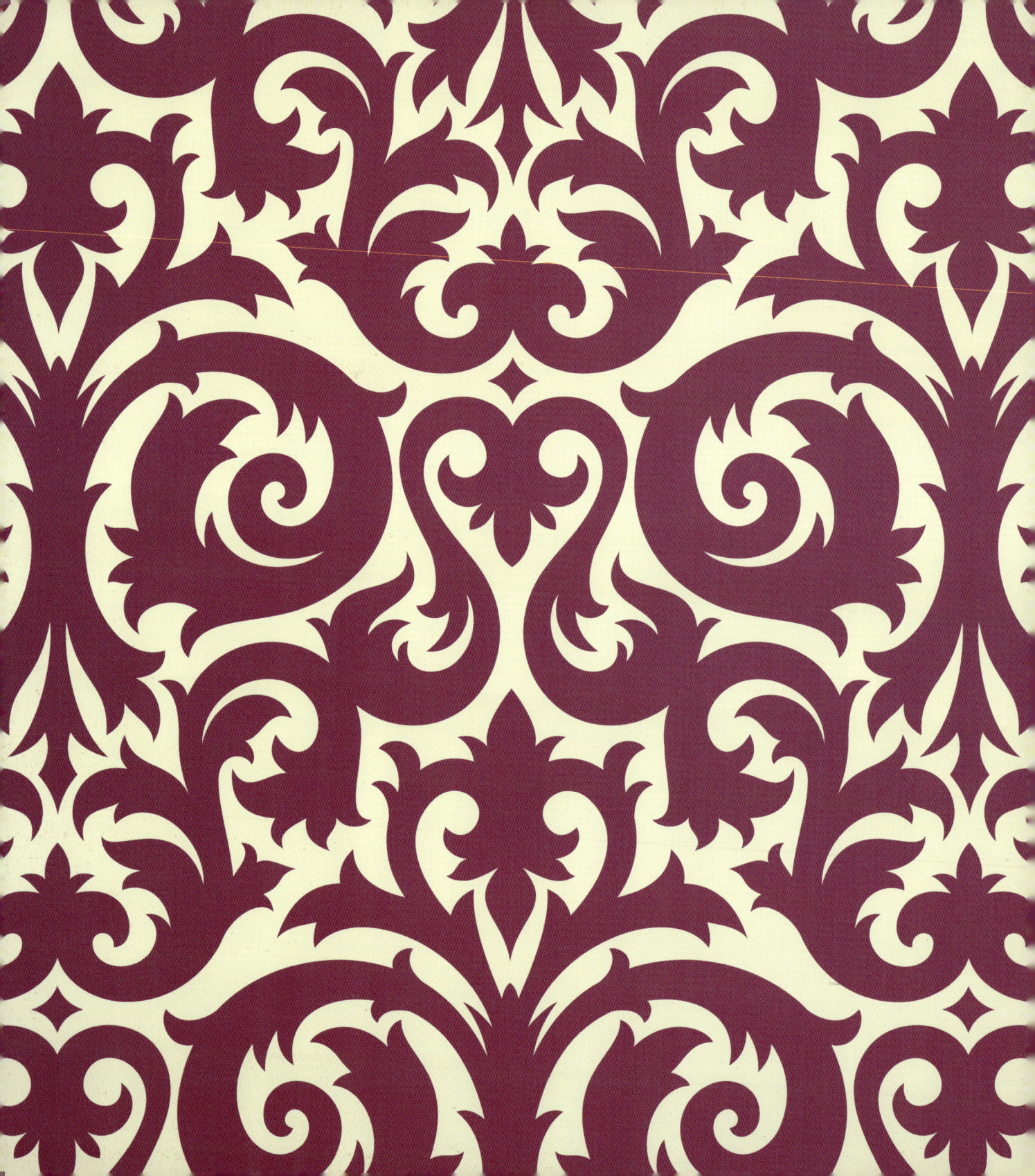

Dessert

Dessert is one of the great pleasures of life, whether it's a slice of lemon meringue pie, or a piece of pav. The fab star rating used in this and the afternoon tea chapters, is different from that used in the other chapters. In the other chapters, the stars refer to the overall nutritional value of the meal but in this chapter, the stars refer to the relative healthiness to the original unhealthy version of the dish. For example, a traditional tiramisu would receive no stars but the fab tiramisu has been given three stars as it so much healthier relative to the traditional fat-filled version.

Often the accompaniment we serve with a dessert is our greatest downfall. So in this chapter, The Finishing Touches (pages 216–217) gives you lots of options for alternatives to a dollop of cream or a scoop of ice-cream, that will not break your nutrition budget.

Managing your sweet tooth can be challenging, so here are some ideas to help you:

Less is more: Often a taste will satisfy a craving without having to have a whole serve. Make mini versions of your favourite desserts, and if you are eating out, share or order something small.

Use your appetite to your advantage: Don't order or think about dessert until 10 minutes after you have finished your main meal. By which time you may be too full to fit one in.

Opt for the naturally low-fat, fruit-based desserts: This includes soufflé, gelato and sorbet. Don't have any cream or ice-cream on the side. Just using this trick will save you lots of calories.

Check the nutrition labels: If you are choosing low-fat desserts at the supermarket, keep an eye on the sugar as some brands use sugar to fill the flavour gap left by the reduced fat.

Use natural sweeteners: Pure maple syrup and fruit juice concentrates offer more than just sugar.

Adapt to lower sugar: Take some time to retrain your tastebuds to like less sweet food.

Have a fruit side: If you are not having a fruit-based dessert, have fresh fruit on the side.

Make dessert a special occasion: Have fresh fruit most nights and leave dessert for special treats.

Blueberry Cheesecake

This cheesecake uses low-fat cream cheese, sponge finger biscuits and a small amount of low-fat spread for the base. Although there is no butter, the flavour is not compromised at all and the fat figure falls from over 40 grams per serve to just 7 grams.

Serves: 10 • **Makes:** 1 cheesecake • **Difficulty:** easy • **Takes:** 20 minutes to prep, 35–40 minutes to cook, plus 2 hours in the fridge

8–10 (170g) sponge finger biscuits

70g good quality spread, melted

1 cup (250g) low-fat or light cream cheese

1 egg

½ cup (115g) caster sugar

2 tablespoons plain flour

1 teaspoon lemon zest

⅔ cup (160ml) light evaporated milk

1 cup (125g) fresh or frozen blueberries

2 teaspoons caster sugar, extra

½ teaspoon cornflour

Set the oven at 180°C.

Crush the sponge fingers to fine crumbs. Place the crumbs in a bowl and pour on the melted spread. Mix together well and then spread over the base of a 23cm springform cake tin. Refrigerate until set.

Beat the cream cheese, egg, caster sugar, plain flour and zest until smooth. Add the evaporated milk and combine well. Fold in ½ cup of the blueberries. Pour the mixture over the set cheesecake crust and smooth out to make it even. Bake for 30–35 minutes, or until set.

Remove the cheesecake from the oven and cool. Refrigerate for 2 hours before serving.

To make the blueberry sauce, place the remaining blueberries in a small saucepan with the extra caster sugar and 3 teaspoons of water and cook until the blueberries begin to release their juice.

Mix the cornflour into a paste with a teaspoon of water and then add to the sauce. Stir until the sauce becomes glossy and thickens. Cool and then refrigerate. If it thickens too much after refrigeration, add a small amount of water to thin it. Just before serving, pour the sauce over the cheesecake.

For a food nerd: Rather than just blueberries, you could use a mix of berries and so further add variety to the dessert. Mixed berries are packed with antioxidants, making them a great choice in any healthy diet. Replace some of the sugar with pure maple syrup or honey.

1 Serve: 7g total fat • 3g saturated fat • 1365kJ (325 calories) • 17g carbohydrates • 5g protein • 1g fibre

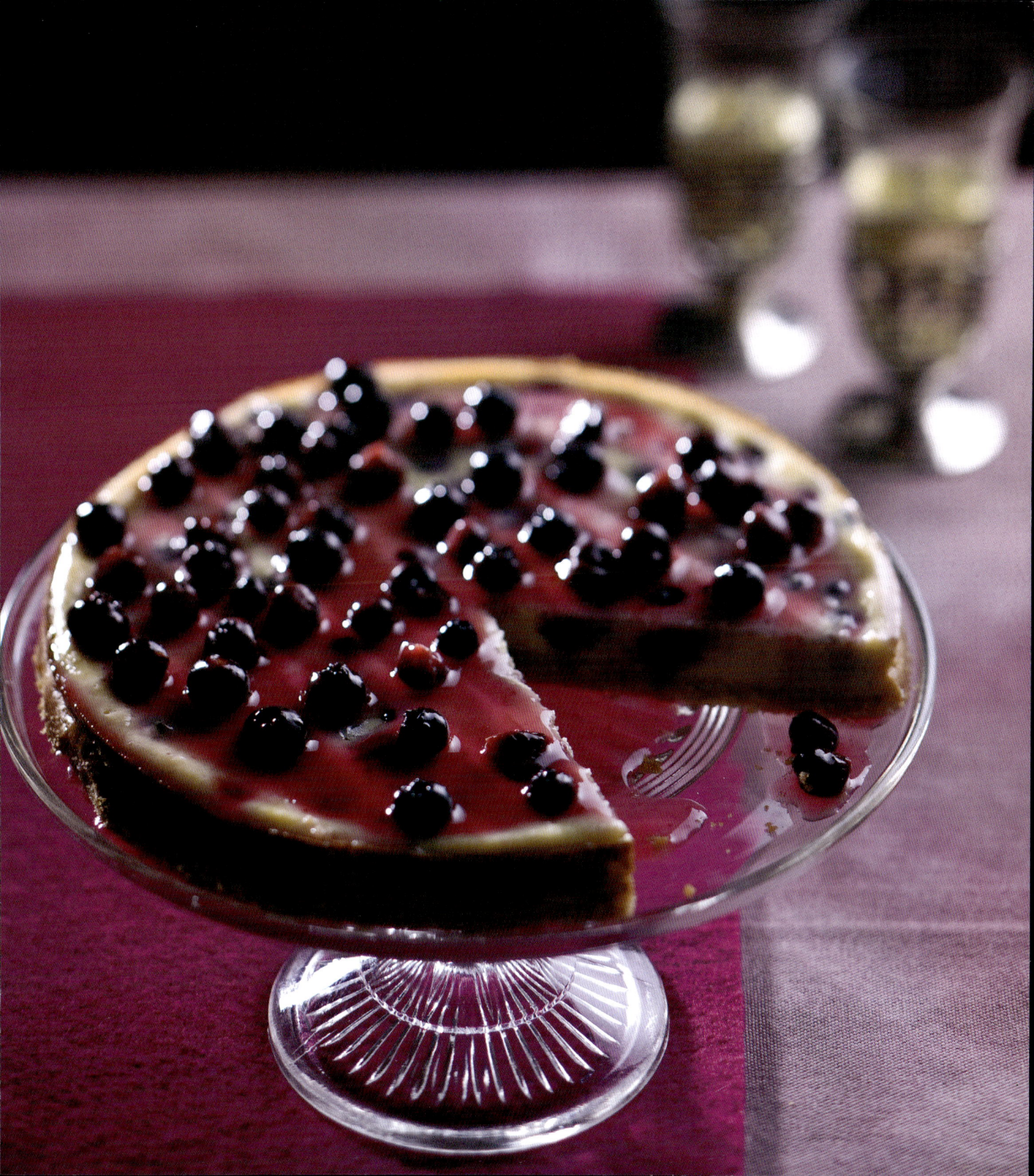

Lemon Cheesecake

By reducing the butter in the crust and the fat in the cheese, you have a fab cheesecake. This scrumptious cheesecake recipe uses a blend of low-fat ricotta and cream cheese, minimal added sugar and has no crumble base, all of which significantly reduces the saturated fat content.

Serves: 10 • **Makes**: 1 cheesecake • **Difficulty**: easy • **Takes**: 15 minutes to prep, 30–35 minutes to cook

65g low-fat natural yoghurt

65g light-cream cheese

1 cup (250g) low-fat or extra-light ricotta cheese

1½ tablespoons grated lemon zest

3 teaspoons plum jam

⅓ cup (40g) plain flour

2 eggs, separated

2 tablespoons caster sugar

Apple and Blackcurrant Jelly Topping (optional)

1 cup (250ml) apple and blackcurrant juice

1½ teaspoons powdered gelatine

Set the oven at 180°C.

Combine the yoghurt, cream cheese, ricotta, lemon zest, plum jam, flour and 1 of the egg yolks in a bowl. Whisk until smooth.

In another bowl, beat the egg whites to soft peaks with an electric mixer. Gradually beat in the sugar until the mixture is glossy and thick. If you take a small amount of the mixture and rub it between your fingers, you should not be able to feel any grittiness from the sugar. This is the best indication that the sugar is dissolved and the whipped egg-sugar mix is ready to use.

Fold the yoghurt ricotta mixture into the beaten egg whites. Gently pour the mixture into a lined 18cm baking-paper springform cake tin. Bake for 30–35 minutes or until set.

Serve with berry compote (page 214) spooned into the centre of the cheesecake or with the apple and blackcurrant jelly topping and sliced fresh fruit in the centre.

To make the apple and blackcurrant jelly topping, heat the juice in a saucepan until hot. Sprinkle the powdered gelatine over the hot juice and stir with a fork to remove any lumps and dissolve the gelatine. Place in the fridge for 30 minutes, or until the jelly has only just begun to set but will still pour. Gently pour enough jelly over the chilled cheesecake to cover the top with a thin film of jelly. Place in the refrigerator and allow to set completely.

1 Serve: 1g total fat • 0.3g saturated fat • 286kJ (68 calories) • 10g carbohydrates • 5g protein • 0.1g fibre

Peach Cobbler

This fruit-and-cake dessert has less butter and sugar than the traditional version and it has been boosted in fibre. Crème Anglaise or custard (page 213) is a great accompaniment to this dessert.

Serves: 8 • **Makes:** 1 pie • **Difficulty:** easy • **Takes:** 15 minutes to prep, 25 minutes to cook

820g tin peach slices in natural juice, drained and roughly chopped

½ cup (75g) wholemeal self-raising flour

½ cup (60g) self-raising flour

¼ cup (55g) raw sugar

1 teaspoon ground cinnamon

50g good quality spread

1 egg

50ml light evaporated milk or low-fat milk

Set the oven at 180°C.

Arrange the peaches in a 23cm pie dish.

In a bowl, combine the flours, sugar and cinnamon.

Rub the spread into the mixture with your fingertips until it is crumbly. Add the egg and just enough milk to make a sticky dough.

Drop the dough roughly over the fruit and spread it so that it covers the peaches. Bake, uncovered for 25 minutes, or until golden brown.

Serve with faux cream (page 217), quick cream (page 216) or low-fat vanilla yoghurt.

1 Serve: 3.5g total fat • 1g saturated fat • 743kJ (177 calories) • 30g carbohydrates • 3g protein • 2g fibre

Lemon Meringue Pot Pies

Pastry, butter, lemon, cream and meringue work together to make a lemon meringue pie. This version uses no pastry, instead it makes individual pot pies in cups. The butter in the lemon cream has been replaced by low-fat spread, further nipping and tucking the delicious pot pies. These are best eaten on the day they are baked.

Serves: 8 • **Makes:** 8 pot pies • **Difficulty:** medium • **Takes:** 15 minutes to prep, 10 minutes to cook

Lemon filling
¼ cup (30g) plain flour
¼ cup (30g) cornflour
¾ cup (165g) raw sugar
¾ cup (185ml) lemon juice
1½ tablespoons lemon zest
1¼ (310ml) cups water
4 egg yolks, lightly beaten
25g good quality spread

Meringue
4 egg whites
3 tablespoons caster sugar

Set the oven at 200°C.

To make the lemon filling, place the flour, cornflour, sugar, lemon juice and zest into a small saucepan, and combine. Over a medium heat, gradually add the water, stirring constantly and cook for 34 minutes until the mixture thickens. Remove from heat and whisk in the egg yolks and spread. Once completely combined, return to the heat and, stirring constantly, cook over low heat for 3–4 minutes, or until it is very thick and glossy.

Evenly divide the mixture between eight ½ cup ramekins.

To make the meringue, use an electric mixer to beat the egg whites until stiff. While still beating, gradually add the caster sugar. Rub a small amount of the meringue mixture between 2 fingers. If there is no gritty feeling from the sugar, then the meringue is ready. If you can still feel the sugar between your fingers, continue beating.

Spoon the meringue on top of the lemon filling in each ramekin. Use a knife to make peaks on the meringue.

Bake for 5–7 minutes, or until the meringue slightly colours on top of the peaks.

1 Serve: 3g total fat • 1g saturated fat • 626kJ (149 calories) • 28.5g carbohydrates • 4g protein • 0g fibre

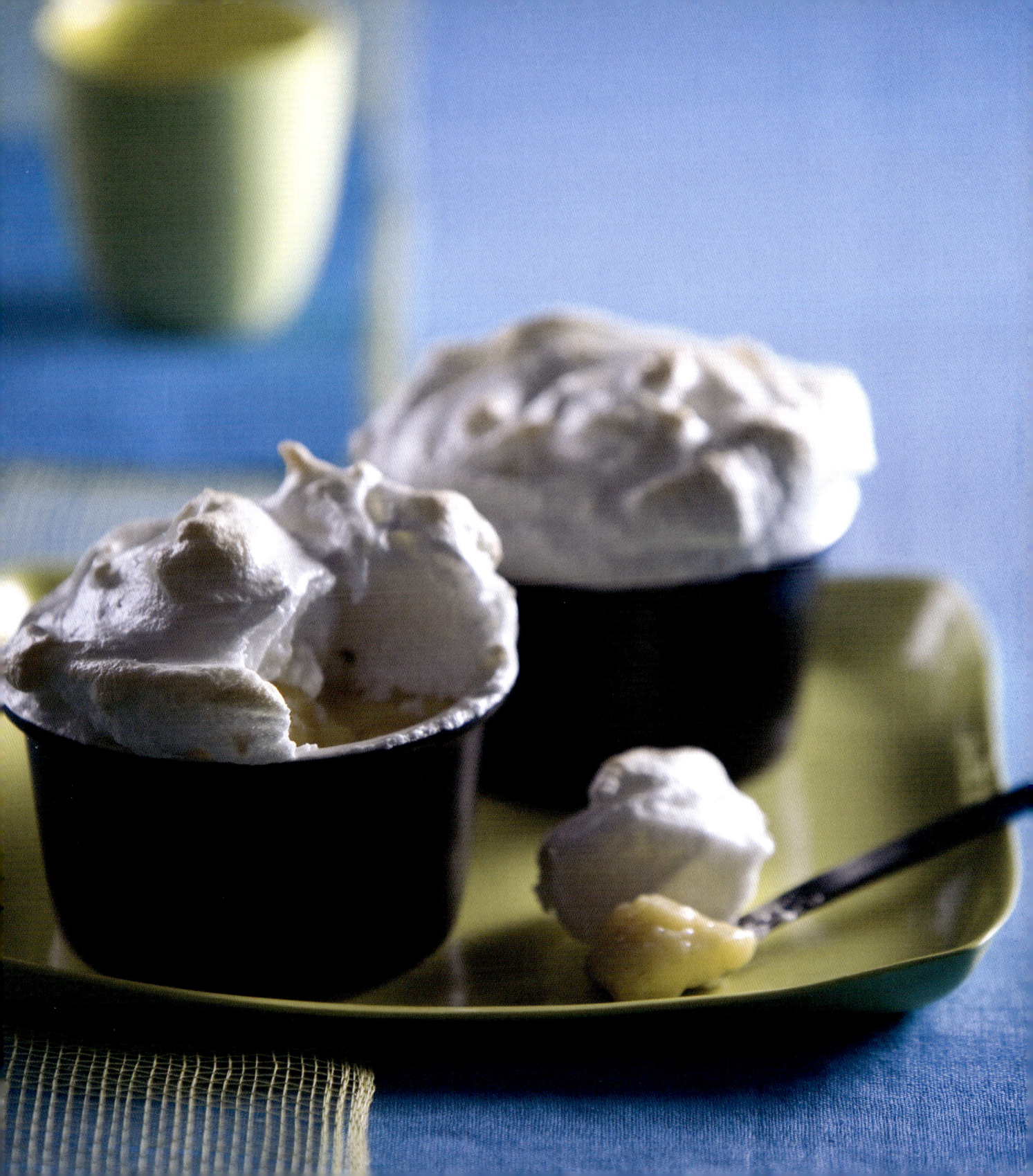

Rich-Baked Custard

This tastes decadent but the creaminess comes from just two eggs and the evaporated milk. Using freshly grated nutmeg makes it even more flavoursome.

Serves: 6 • **Difficulty:** easy • **Takes:** 5 minutes to prep, 30-40 minutes to cook

2 eggs

1½ tablespoons raw sugar

1 tablespoon pure maple syrup

3 drops natural vanilla extract

1½ cups (375ml) low-fat evaporated milk

½ teaspoon ground or freshly grated nutmeg

Set the oven at 180°C.

Beat the eggs, sugar and maple syrup lightly. Add the vanilla.

Warm the milk in a saucepan until foam just begins to appear on the side of the pan, then slowly add it to the egg and sugar mixture and mix well.

Pour into a 1-litre ovenproof dish or into individual ramekins. Sprinkle with the nutmeg.

Stand the dish or the ramekins in a large baking pan. Fill the pan with boiling water to come halfway up the side of the dish or the ramekins. Place the pan in the oven.

Bake for 35–40 minutes, or until the custard is just set in the centre. The custard should still slightly wobble when removed from the oven as it will continue cooking as it cools.

Serving suggestion: Serve with tinned fruit, sliced banana or stone fruit in season.

1 Serve: 2.5g total fat • 1g saturated fat • 428kJ (102 calories) • 14g carbohydrates • 7g protein • 0g fibre

Vanilla Panna Cotta

Panna cotta is cream set with gelatine and delivers a hefty 34 grams of fat per serve. Using naturally thick and creamy Greek yoghurt in this recipe gives you the feeling and taste of the richness of cream without the fat and kilojoules.

Serves: 4 • **Makes:** 4 panna cottas • **Difficulty:** easy • **Takes:** 15 minutes to prep

1½ teaspoons powdered gelatine

1 tablespoon caster sugar

⅔ cup (160ml) skim milk

300g low-fat natural or no-fat Greek yoghurt

½ teaspoons natural vanilla extract

In a small saucepan, sprinkle the gelatine and sugar over the milk and heat gently. Do not allow to boil. Remove from the heat when the sugar and gelatine have dissolved. Allow to cool slightly.

Combine the yoghurt and vanilla in a bowl. Slowly add the cooled milk mixture to the yoghurt mixture and combine well.

Pour into jelly moulds and place in the refrigerator until they are set.

Serve in the jelly moulds or run a wet knife around the rim and turn the panna cottas onto serving plates and serve with fresh fruit.

1 Serve: 1g total fat • 0g saturated fat • 269kJ (64 calories) • 8g carbohydrates • 8g protein • 0g fibre

Tiramisu

Tiramisu contains the king of all creams, mascarpone. It is technically a cheese but, in cooking, it is used like cream and has the fat content of a double or triple cream, that is 60–75 per cent. It is a central ingredient in traditional tiramisu where it is layered with chocolate, biscuits, brandy and espresso coffee. In this version, mascarpone is replaced by a blend of cream cheese, low-fat ricotta and skim milk, and is layered in a glass rather than a large bowl. So it looks beautiful, makes sure you only have a limited serving and cuts those nasty saturated fats down from 26 grams to only 1 gram per serve.

Serves: 4 • **Makes**: 4 • **Difficulty**: easy • **Takes**: 15 minutes to prep, plus 2 hours in fridge

⅓ cup (90g) light-cream cheese
⅓ cup (90g) low-fat or no-fat ricotta cheese
½ teaspoon natural vanilla extract
2 tablespoons skim milk
2 tablespoons icing sugar
8 sponge finger biscuits
1 cup (125ml) espresso coffee, cooled
2 squares of dark chocolate, grated

Beat together the cream cheese, ricotta, vanilla, milk and icing sugar in a bowl.

Break the sponge fingers into chunks and quickly dip them into the coffee, then divide a third of them between four fancy glasses or parfait glasses. Spoon a dollop of the cheese mix over the fingers. Repeat the layers of sponge fingers and cheese mix until the glasses are full. Top with a teaspoonful of the grated dark chocolate.

Cover with cling film and refrigerate for a couple of hours to allow the flavours to meld.

For a food nerd: Add a layer of fresh fruit like sliced banana, strawberries or blueberries.

1 Serve: 2g total fat • 1g saturated fat • 554kJ (132 calories) • 11g carbohydrates • 6g protein • 1g fibre

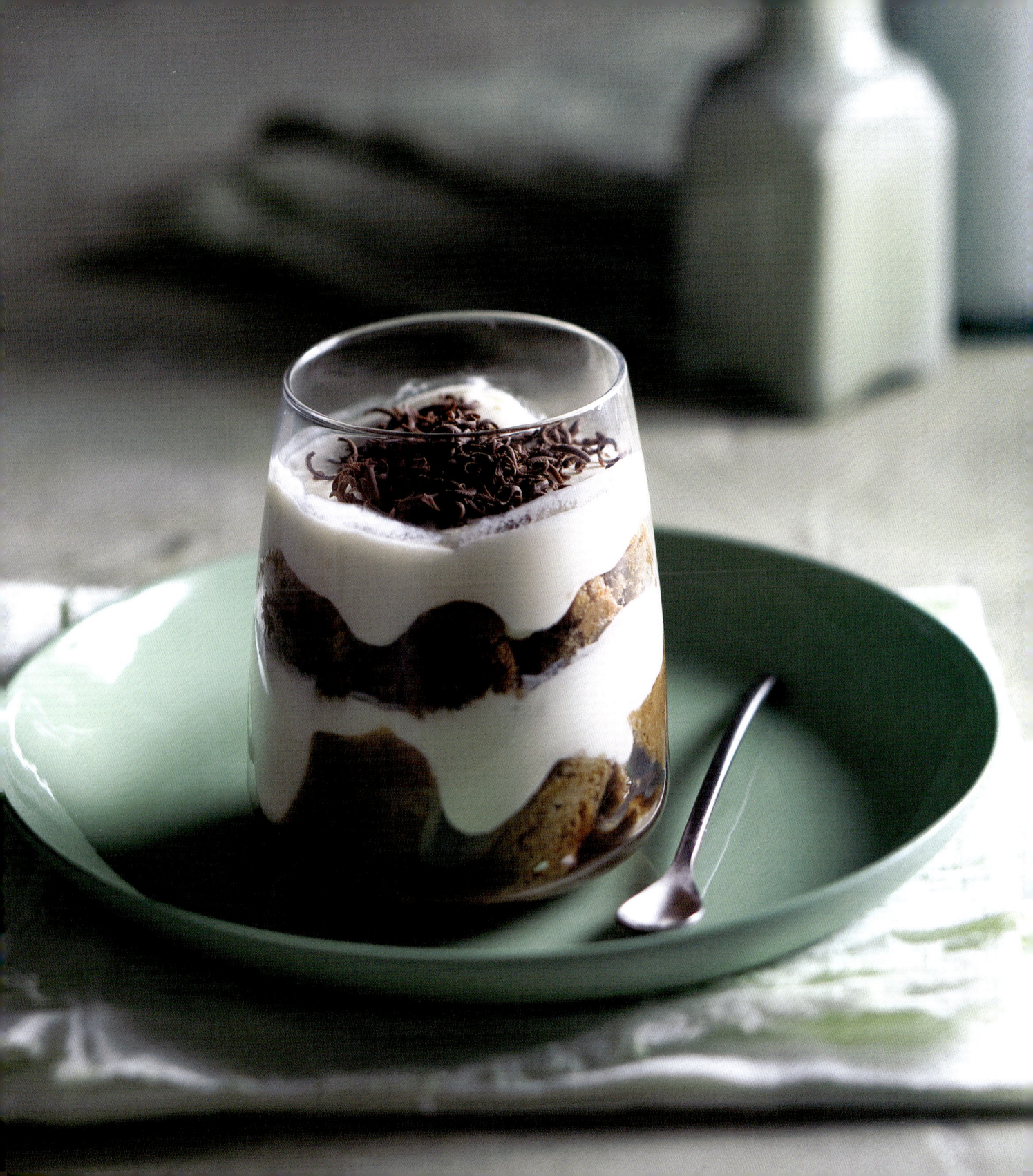

Crème Brûlée

Like crème caramel, this dessert is usually filled with cream, eggs and over 50 grams of fat! There is no cream in this version, keeping it low in saturated fat.

Serves: 6 • **Makes:** 6 crème brûlée • **Difficulty:** medium • **Takes:** 30 minutes to prep, 35 minutes to cook, 4 hours in the fridge

2 cups (500ml) low-fat evaporated milk

1 teaspoon natural vanilla extract

½ cup (115g) caster sugar

3 eggs

2 egg whites

2 tablespoons caster sugar, extra

Set the oven at 150°C.

Combine the evaporated milk, vanilla and half of the caster sugar in a saucepan over medium heat. Stir to dissolve the sugar, then slowly bring to the boil. Remove from the heat as soon as it begins to boil.

Whisk the eggs and egg whites with the remaining sugar in a bowl. Slowly add the hot milk to the eggs, whisking all the time. Ladle or pour the mix into six 8cm ramekins.

Bake for 30–35 minutes, or until just set but still wobbly in the centre. Cool, then refrigerate for 1–2 hours.

Remove the ramekins from the fridge about 20 minutes before serving. Sprinkle the extra caster sugar over each crème brûlée and place under a hot grill for 3 minutes, or until the sugar on top caramelises and is golden. Carefully remove from the grill.

Serve.

1 Serve: 3.5g total fat • 1.6g saturated fat • 743kJ (177 calories) • 27g carbohydrates • 11g protein • 0g fibre

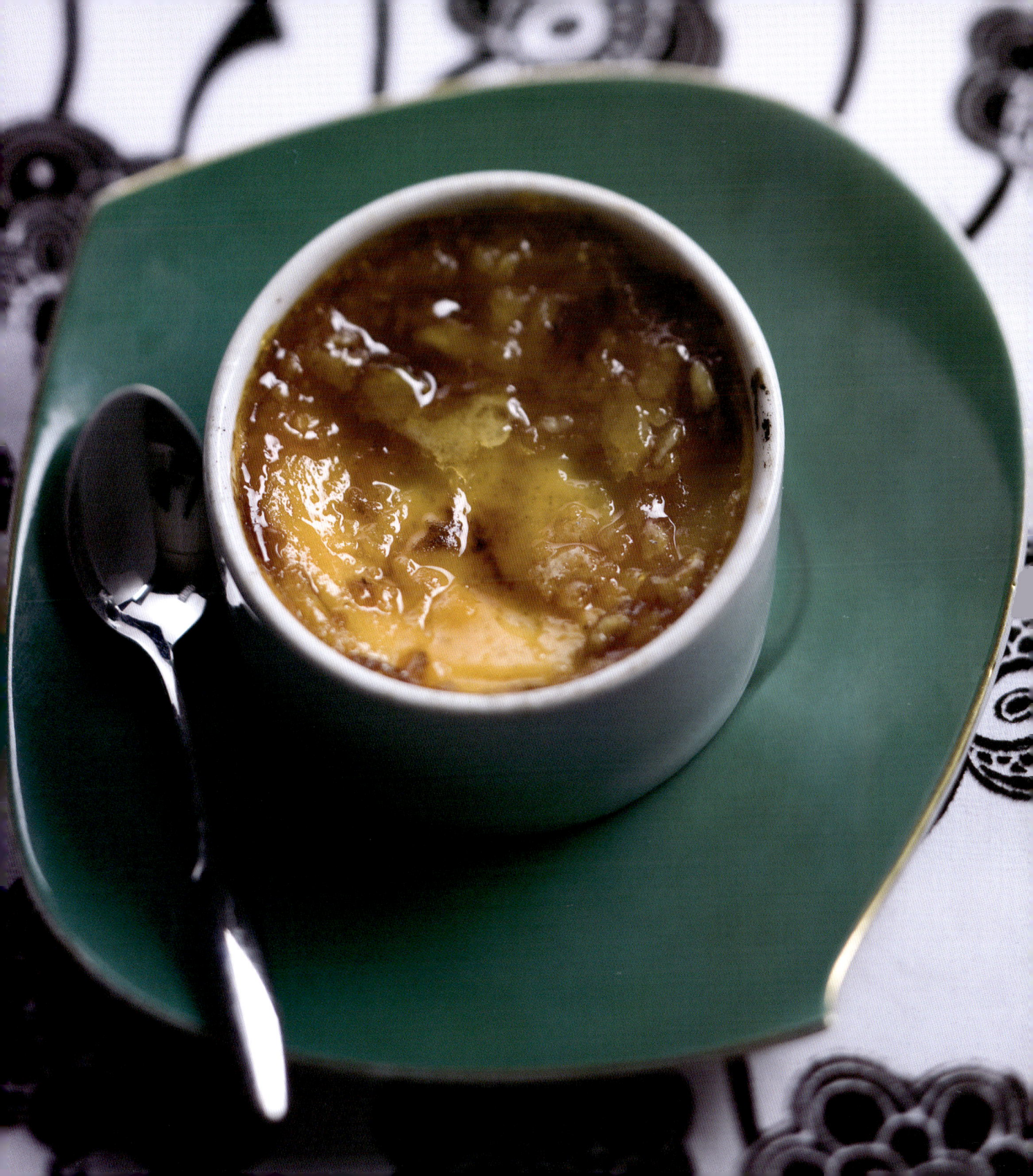

Crème Caramel

You won't find any of the usual double cream or extra egg yolks in this crème caramel recipe but you will still find the delectable caramel taste. The trick with making a crème caramel is to take it out of the oven just before the centre is set so that the residual heat continues to cook it.

Serves: 4 • **Makes:** 4 caramels • **Difficulty:** medium • **Takes:** 30 minutes to prep, 20 minutes to cook, plus chilling time

⅔ cup (140g) sugar
⅓ cup (80ml) water
1 teaspoon natural vanilla extract
4 eggs, lightly beaten
⅓ cup (80g) caster sugar
2 cups (500ml) low-fat evaporated milk

Set the oven at 200°C.

Put the sugar and water in a small saucepan over a low heat. Stir for 2–3 minutes, or until the sugar dissolves. Turn the heat up to medium and bring to the boil. Use a wet pastry brush to brush any sugar crystals off the side of the pan during the boiling process so they don't burn. Be really careful as it is incredibly hot. Continue boiling, without stirring for 8–10 minutes, or until the toffee turns a light golden colour. Very carefully divide the toffee between four ramekins. Set aside.

Place the vanilla, eggs and caster sugar in a jug or bowl and beat until well combined.

In a saucepan, slowly bring the milk to boiling point. When it just reaches boiling point, immediately remove from the heat and very slowly whisk the milk into the egg mixture.

Pour the egg and milk mixture over the toffee in the ramekins. Place the ramekins in a baking pan. Fill the pan with boiling water so it comes halfway up the sides of the ramekins to make a water bath.

Bake for 20 minutes, or until the custard is nearly set in the centre.

When cooked, chill the crème caramels for a minimum of 3 hours, then run a knife around the inner edge of the ramekins and turn out the crème caramels onto serving plates, toffee side up.

For a food nerd: Reduce the sugar to ½ cup (110g) and only use ¼ cup (60ml) of water for the caramel.

1 Serve: 6g total fat • 3g saturated fat • 1554kJ (370 calories) • 66g carbohydrates • 15g protein • 0g fibre

Jaffa Self-saucing Pudding

This is lovely served with faux cream (page 217).

Serves: 6 • **Difficulty:** easy • **Takes:** 20 minutes to prep, 35–40 minutes to cook

good quality vegetable
  oil cooking spray
50g good quality spread
½ cup (125ml) skim milk
½ teaspoon natural
  vanilla extract
⅔ cup (140g) raw sugar
½ cup (75g) wholemeal
  self-raising flour
½ cup (60g) self-raising
  flour
2 tablespoons
  unsweetened cocoa
  powder
zest of 1 orange
½ cup (115g) firmly
  packed brown sugar
1½ cups (375ml) boiling
  water

Set the oven at 180°C.

Lightly spray a 23cm pudding basin with the oil.

Melt the spread in a saucepan, then remove the pan from heat. Add the milk and vanilla. Set aside.

Combine the raw sugar, flours, 1 tablespoon of cocoa and the zest in a bowl. Add the milk-and-spread mixture and stir well. Pour into the pudding basin.

Sift the remaining cocoa powder and the brown sugar over the pudding. Gently pour the water over the back of a metal spoon (so it doesn't dent the cake mixture) onto the pudding.

Bake for 35–40 minutes, or until the top is firm to the touch.

For a food nerd: Reduce the raw sugar to ½ cup (110g).

1 Serve: 4g total fat • 1g saturated fat • 1067kJ (254 calories) • 52g carbohydrates • 3g protein • 0.3g fibre

Bread and Butter Pudding

Cream, butter and egg yolks are a big part of the traditional bread and butter pudding with 50 grams of fat per serve, 28 grams of which are saturated, it desperately needs a makeover. Light or low-fat evaporated milk replaces the cream beautifully in this recipe, but unlike the cream, it doesn't hang around on the hips …

Serves: 6 • **Makes:** 6 serves • **Difficulty:** easy • **Takes:** 10 minutes to prep, 40 minutes to cook

good quality vegetable oil cooking spray

1 small French stick, cut into chunky slices

2 tablespoon good quality spread

½ cup (60g) sultanas

185ml tin low-fat evaporated milk

1½ cups (325ml) skim or low-fat milk

1 egg

2 egg whites

2 teaspoons natural vanilla extract

2 teaspoons ground nutmeg

½ cup (110g) raw sugar

Set the oven to 180°C.

Spray a 20cm shallow ovenproof dish with the oil.

Cover one side of each slice of bread with some of the spread.

Place the bread, spread side up, in the prepared dish. Sprinkle the sultanas over the bread.

In a bowl, whisk together the evaporated milk, skim milk, egg, egg whites, vanilla, nutmeg and sugar. Pour the custard mixture over the bread.

Bake for 40 minutes, or until golden brown and set.

For a food nerd: Use high-fibre wholemeal bread and cut down on the sugar, but increase the amount of sultanas a little if you need to boost the sweetness.

1 **Serve:** 3g total fat • 1g saturated fat • 853kJ (203 calories) • 28g carbohydrates • 7.5g protein • 0.4g fibre

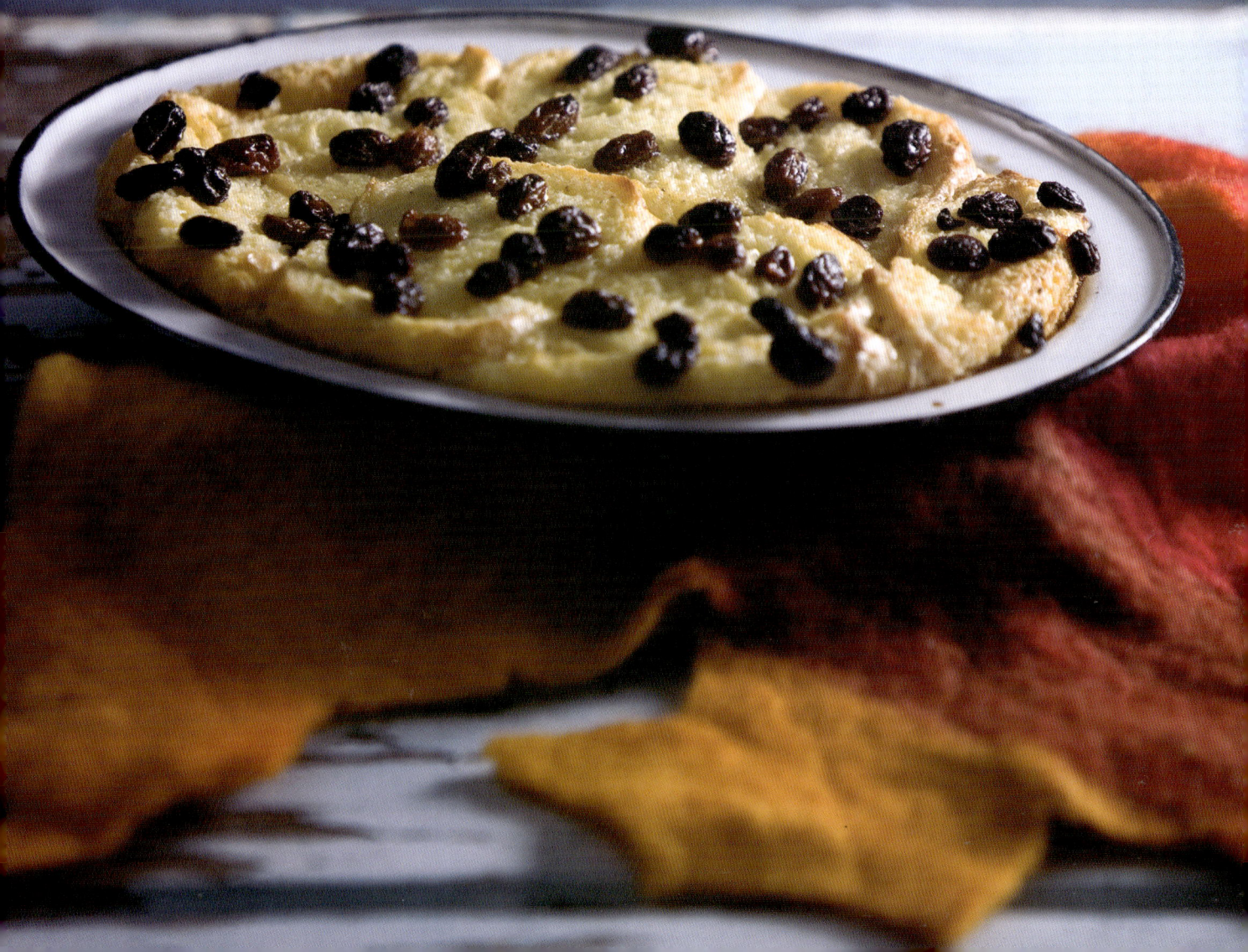

Apple Pie

It is the pastry that makes traditional apple pie a fat recipe. This recipe uses 25% reduced-fat puff pastry and less by covering the apple filling with strips of pastry in a lattice pattern. You must use just the right amount of water so that when the apples are stewed they do not need to be drained. If you drain them, you lose lots of nutrients down the sink with the water.

Serves: 8 • **Makes:** 1 apple pie • **Difficulty:** easy • **Takes:** 30 minutes to prep, 30 minutes to cook

7 granny smith apples, peeled, cored and sliced
2 tablespoons raw sugar
2 whole cloves
1–2 tablespoons water
2 sheets 25% reduced-fat puff pastry
½ teaspoon melted good quality spread

Set the oven at 200°C.

Place apples, sugar, cloves and water into a large saucepan, cover with a lid and gently simmer until the apples are translucent and soft (about 10 minutes). Remove from heat.

Line a 23cm pie dish with one sheet of the puff pastry. Trim the edges to fit the dish. Using a fork, prick some holes in the pastry.

Place a sheet of baking paper over the pastry and cover the paper with a cupful of baking beads, dried beans or rice. Place in the oven and blind bake (see 'Cooking tips', page 241, for directions) until the pastry is lightly browned. Remove the weights and baking paper.

Spoon the apples into the pastry shell.

Cut the second sheet of pastry into 2cm strips. Arrange the strips over the pie in a lattice design. This is for effect, so use only a few strips and don't attempt to cover the entire top of the pie.

Lightly brush the pastry with the melted spread.

Bake for 10 minutes, then reduce the temperature to 180°C and bake for a further 20 minutes, or until the pastry is golden.

Serving suggestions: Serve with faux cream (page 217) or low-fat vanilla yoghurt.

For a food nerd: To further reduce the pastry and fat content of this dessert, use a simple meringue on top in place of the pastry. It looks fantastic.

1 Serve: 3g total fat • 1g saturated fat • 1394kJ (332 calories) • 27g carbohydrates • 1g protein • 3g fibre

Pear Crumble

Butter is one of the things that gives crumble its crunchy crumble effect. Here the crunch comes from a reduced amount of good quality spread. The nutrition has been boosted by the addition of sunflower seeds and cashews.

Serves: 6 • **Difficulty:** easy • **Takes:** 10 minutes to prep, 20 minutes to cook

⅓ cup (80g) packed brown sugar

¼ teaspoon ground nutmeg

½ teaspoon ground cinnamon

⅔ cup (65g) rolled oats

⅓ cup (30g) wheat germ

1 tablespoon chopped cashews

1 tablespoon sunflower seeds

2 tablespoons melted good quality spread

400g tin pears in natural juice, drained and diced

Set the oven at 180°C.

Mix all the dry ingredients together.

Add the melted spread to the dry ingredients and mix until it resembles breadcrumbs.

Arrange the diced pears in the base of a 23cm pie dish.

Spoon the crumble mix on top of the fruit.

Bake for 20 minutes, or until the crumble is browned and the fruit is bubbling.

1 Serve: 4.5g total fat • 0.6g saturated fat • 680kJ (162 calories) • 30g carbohydrates • 3g protein • 2.8g fibre

Sticky Date Pudding

This pudding has had the fab treatment with a reduction in sugar and fat, and a boost in fibre. Looking at the nutrition panel, you will see that even the fab version of this pud still has 13 grams of fat (down from its pre-makeover of 41 grams), so keep this one for special occasions.

Serves: 6 • **Makes:** 6 small puddings • **Difficulty:** easy • **Takes:** 15 minutes to prep, 25 minutes to cook

good quality vegetable oil
  cooking spray
1 cup (180g) roughly chopped
  pitted dates
½ cup (125ml) water
½ cup (60g) self-raising flour
½ cup (75g) wholemeal self-
  raising flour
½ cup (95g) firmly packed brown
  sugar
2 eggs
1 teaspoon natural vanilla extract
⅓ cup (80ml) sunflower, nut or
  olive oil

Butterscotch sauce
1 teaspoon cornflour
147ml tin low-fat evaporated milk
⅓ cup (80g) firmly packed brown
  sugar
30g good quality spread
50ml low-fat milk

Set the oven at 180°C.

Lightly spray 6 ovenproof coffee cups with the oil. Cut out six circles of baking paper to line the base of each coffee cup.

Place the dates and water in a small saucepan. Bring to the boil, then remove from heat and cool. Drain the dates.

Sift the flours into a bowl, then add the brown sugar, drained dates, the eggs, vanilla and oil. Combine well. Pour the mixture into the prepared cups.

Bake for 25 minutes, or until the puddings are cooked in the centre.

To make the sauce, mix the cornflour with 2 tablespoons of the evaporated milk to make a smooth paste. Set aside.

In a small saucepan, combine the sugar, spread, remaining evaporated milk and low-fat milk. Simmer gently for 5 minutes. Add the cornflour paste and cook, stirring, for a further 2–3 minutes, or until it begins to thicken.

When the puddings are ready, poke holes in the top of them and pour a tablespoon of sauce into each. Return the puddings to the oven for a further 5 minutes.

Bring the remaining sauce to the boil, reduce heat and simmer, stirring constantly, until the sauce thickens slightly and coats the back of a wooden spoon. Remove from heat.

Take the puddings from the oven and turn out onto serving plates and pour some sauce over each pudding.

Serving suggestons: Serve with faux cream (page 217), quick cream (page 216) or low-fat vanilla yoghurt.

1 Serve: 13g total fat • 2.4g saturated fat • 1701kJ (405 calories) • 67g carbohydrates • 7g protein • 2.4g fibre

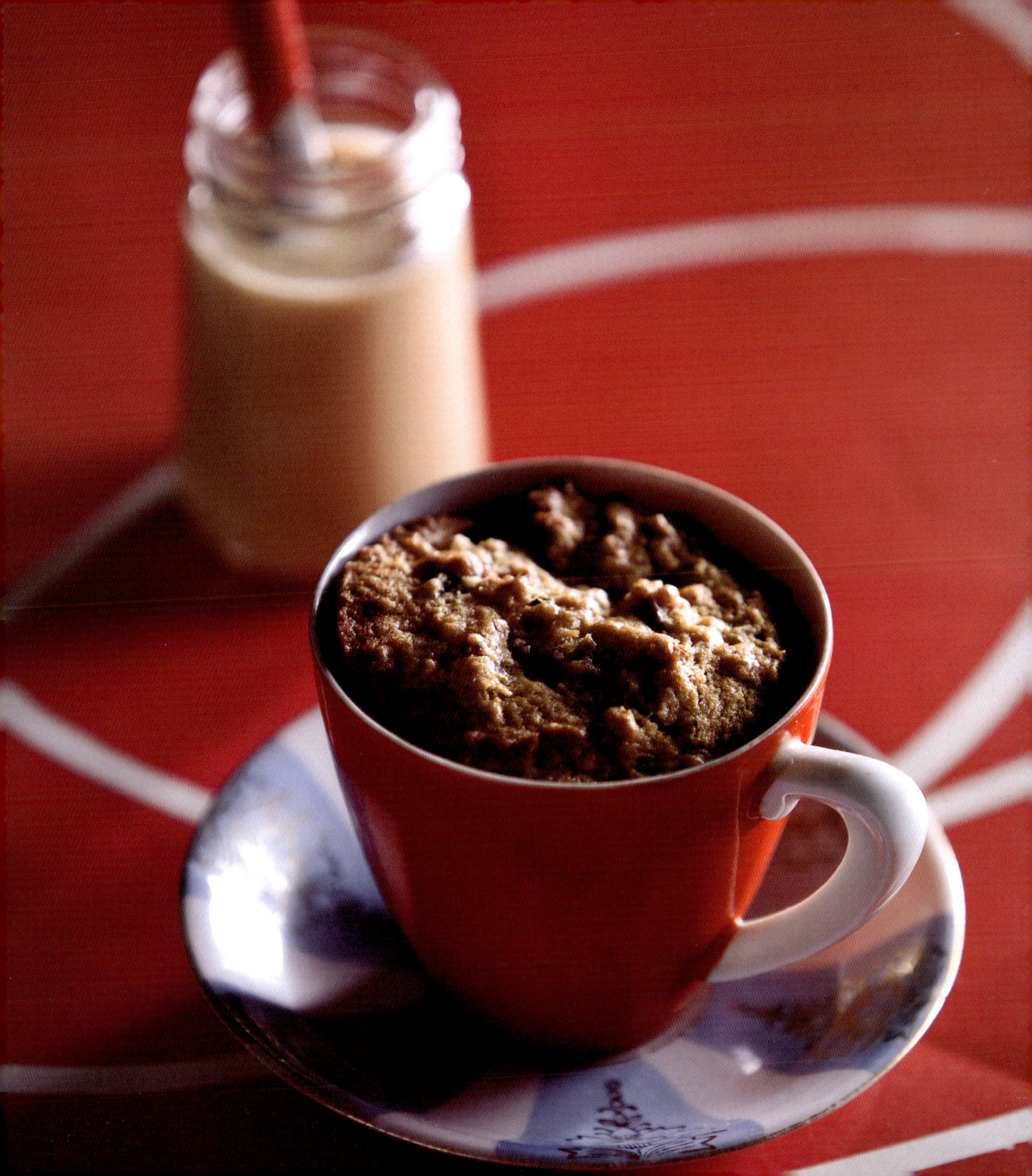

A handy guide to portion

Whether you are heavy or slim, overeating is not a good option and will undermine your healthy eating makeover. How much you eat is just as important as considering what you eat, so here is a toolbox to help you get some portion perspective.

The portion toolbox

Your hand

Your *palm* shows the size of your serve of protein and the thickness of your palm indicates how thick the portion should be.

Your *closed fist* shows how big your serve of starchy carbohydrates should be.

The size of both *cupped hands* shows the amount of vegetables and salad you should have on your plate.

One cupped hand shows the amount of green vegetables you should have.

The *tip of your thumb* is the maximum amount of sugar or added fat or low-fat mayonnaise you can add if you feel you need these with your meal.

Your plate

Use only standard 25cm dinner plates. Larger plates will lead to larger meals. If you are having dessert, have it in a teacup. It keeps your serve small and looks great too.

Your patience

Time is a critical factor in controlling portion. Give your stomach 10 minutes to tell you if you really *need* seconds. After a ten-minute wait, chances are you will be full, and saying no to seconds will be easy.

Your danger times and triggers

Know your danger times: they may be 3 o'clock in the afternoon, straight after work or while you are preparing dinner. Work out something you can do to distract yourself to get through these times or have some small, divided portions of healthy options available. If you are ravenous as soon as you walk through the door in the evening, have a large glass of water and a piece of fruit before you reach for anything else. If you can't help picking while you are preparing dinner, keep some serving-sized containers of homemade vegetable soup in the freezer and defrost a mug of soup to have. This will help to ease your hunger pangs and also add to your fibre and nutrient intake for the day.

Your willpower

Be honest with yourself. If you are lacking in willpower, work that fact into your healthy eating plans. Don't have tempting unhealthy food options in the house; eat just before you go grocery shopping; take a small healthy snack to have with your morning cappuccino so you don't buy a junk snack; plan to indulge your cravings during your RDOs and divide up any treats into individual serving sizes so you are not tempted to eat the whole packet or box.

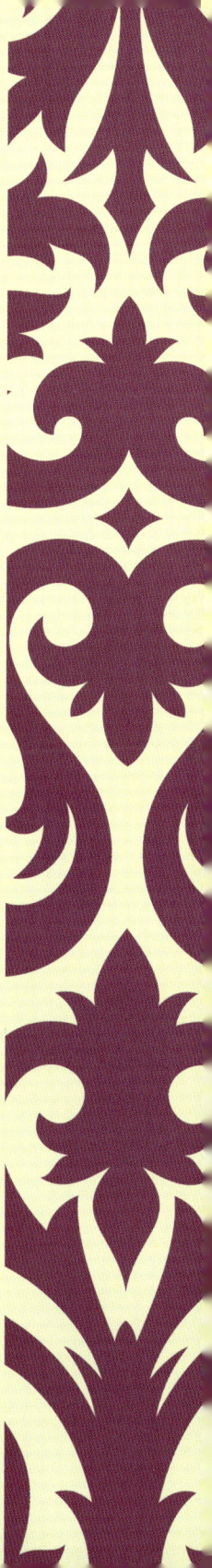

White Chocolate Mousse

A chocolate mousse seems so indulgent but this one is far from being a guilty pleasure. The evaporated milk does all of the work and lends next to no fat. From the fat version's 47 grams of fat per serve, we go down to a fab 2 grams. Perfect!

Serves: 6-8 • **Difficulty:** easy • **Takes:** 20 minutes to prep, plus chilling time

1 tablespoon powdered
  gelatine
⅓ cup (80g) caster sugar
375ml tin low-fat
  evaporated milk,
  chilled
½ cup (85g) chopped
  white chocolate

Sprinkle the gelatine and sugar over 2 tablespoons of water in a small saucepan. Over medium heat, gently dissolve the gelatine and sugar. Remove from heat.

Using an electric mixer, whip the evaporated milk until fluffy (3–5 minutes).

Melt the white chocolate using the microwave or a double saucepan on the stovetop.

If using a microwave, place the chocolate in a microwave-safe bowl, turn the power down to medium, and heat in 20 second bursts, stirring with a wooden spoon between each heating period, until the chocolate has melted. If using the stovetop, put the chocolate into a heatproof glass bowl and place over a saucepan of simmering water. Do not allow the base of the bowl to touch the water. Stir using a wooden spoon or wooden chopstick. Once melted, remove from the heat.

Using an electric mixer, slowly add the gelatine mix then the white chocolate to the whipped milk, while continually beating. When ready, it will look light and fluffy.

Place in a bowl or freezer container, cover and put in the freezer for an hour and then transfer to the fridge until ready to serve.

For a food nerd: Serve with a bowl of fresh seasonal fruit.

1 Serve: 2g total fat • 1g saturated fat • 386kJ (92 calories) • 15g carbohydrates • 4g protein • 0.2g fibre

Strawberry Mousse

This mousse creates a lot of dirty dishes, but it is worth the effort as it is light and fluffy — but contains no cream. It really captures the lovely taste of fresh strawberries. Serve it with fresh fruit, as a component of a parfait.

Serves: 6-8 • **Difficulty:** medium • **Takes:** 20 minutes to prep, plus chilling time

1 tablespoon powdered
  gelatine
¼ cup (55g) caster sugar
1½ cups (200g)
  strawberries, mashed
1½ tablespoons
  strawberry jam
375ml tin low-fat
  evaporated milk,
  chilled

Sprinkle the gelatine and sugar over 2 tablespoons of water in a small saucepan and gently heat until the gelatine and sugar dissolve. Add the mashed strawberries and jam and combine. Remove from heat.

Allow to cool for 5 minutes, then push the mixture through a sieve to remove all the berry seeds. Set aside.

Using an electric mixer, whip the chilled evaporated milk until fluffy (3–5 minutes).

Gently fold the sieved strawberry mixture into the whipped milk. Place in the freezer for an hour (set the timer!) and then transfer to the fridge until ready to serve.

For a food nerd: Serve with a bowl of fresh seasonal berries.

1 Serve: 1g total fat • 0.5g saturated fat • 983kJ (234 calories) • 16.5g carbohydrates • 4g protein • 0.6g fibre

Double Chocolate Strawberries

Chocolate-dipped strawberries are usually dipped in chocolate to just below the hull. A different technique is used with these strawberries. The white and dark chocolate is melted and then drizzled over the strawberries so as to look like a chocolate web. This still gives you the taste (and a beautiful effect) but you only use ⅓ of the chocolate you would use in the traditional chocolate-dipped strawberries.

Makes: 20 chocolate strawberries • **Difficulty**: medium • **Takes**: 10 minutes to prep

2 punnets strawberries, washed and dried*
1 tablespoon (15g) dark chocolate bits (70% cocoa)
1 tablespoon (15g) white chocolate bits

Line a baking tray with baking paper and place the washed and dried strawberries on the tray in a single layer.

Melt the dark and milk chocolate bits separately. If using a microwave, place each chocolate in a microwave-safe glass bowl, turn the power down to medium, and heat in 20-second bursts, stirring with a wooden spoon between each heating until the chocolate has melted. If using the stovetop, put each chocolate in a heatproof glass bowl and place over a saucepan of simmering water. Do not allow the base of the bowl to touch the water as we want the steam to melt the chocolate not the water. Stir using a wooden spoon or wooden chopstick. Once melted, remove from the heat.

Dip a chopstick into the white chocolate and then drizzle the chocolate over the strawberries to create a web effect. You should be able to still see lots of red from the strawberry through the fine chocolate.

Repeat with the dark chocolate.

Allow to set and serve.

* When washing strawberries, always leave the hulls (green bits) on as these prevent the water from penetrating the fruit and making it soggy.

1 **Serve**: 1g total fat • 0.4g saturated fat • 63kJ (15 calories) • 2g carbohydrates • 0.3g protein • 0.6g fibre

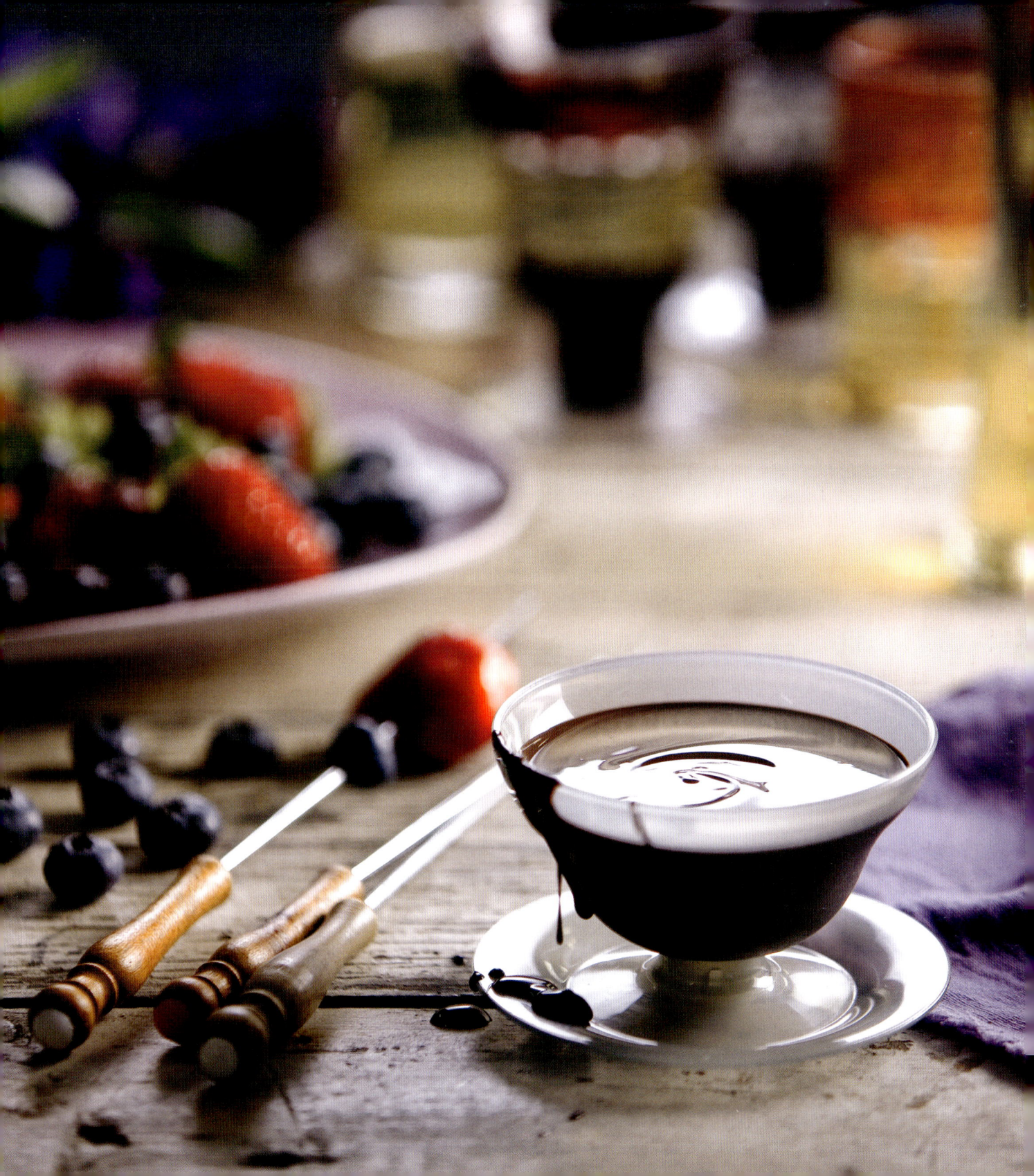

Ivy May's Trifle

I vividly remember my Nanna's trifle. She filled it with cake, sherry, jelly, custard, fresh cream, a couple of slices of fresh fruit and a dash more sherry. Nanna's recipe has had a makeover, which I know she is happy with because I checked! The cream has disappeared, along with the sherry; the jelly is all natural; the custard is low-fat; and there is loads of fresh fruit. You could use low-fat shop-bought custard but first check that the sugar content is low.

Serves: 10 • **Makes:** 1 large trifle • **Difficulty:** easy • **Takes:** 20 minutes to prep, 1 hour to set

8 sponge finger biscuits

1 packet jelly, (natural colours and flavours)

400g tin peach pieces in natural juice, drained

1 quantity custard (page 213)

400g tin pear pieces in natural juice, drained

1 banana, peeled and sliced

4 tablespoons faux cream (page 217) low-fat vanilla yoghurt

1 punnet strawberries, washed, hulled and sliced

Break the sponge fingers into three pieces and line the base of a 20cm glass serving bowl.

Make the jelly as per the directions on the packet. Pour one third of the jelly over the sponge fingers and allow to soak. Place the remaining jelly in the fridge to set.

Put a layer of the peaches on top of the sponge fingers and the set jelly. Then cover the peaches with one-third of the custard. Next add a layer of pears then bananas and cover with more custard. Continue layering until all the fruit and custard is used. Finish with a layer of custard.

Drop spoonfuls of faux cream or vanilla yoghurt over the top of the custard.

Cut the remaining set jelly into cubes and sprinkle over the top of the custard.

Place sliced fresh strawberries on top.

Serve immediately or keep in the fridge until ready to serve.

For a food nerd: Reduce the amount of sugar in the custard as the other trifle ingredients are already sweet.

1 Serve: 1.5g total fat • 0.4g saturated fat • 462kJ (110 calories) • 19g carbohydrates • 2g protein • 2.5g fibre

Banana Split

This banana split has more banana than ice-cream; homemade chocolate sauce instead of preservative-laden shop-bought topping; low-fat ice-cream or yoghurt; whipped milk instead of cream; and almonds instead of peanuts. Nutritionally, almonds are a great source of calcium and are far superior to the crushed peanuts usually used to top a sundae or split.

Serves: 4 • **Makes:** 4 splits • **Difficulty:** easy • **Takes:** 10 minutes to prep

¼ cup (80g) almonds

4 ripe bananas, peeled

½ cup (125ml) full-fat evaporated milk, chilled

8 tablespoons homemade banana ice-cream (page 212) or low-fat vanilla ice-cream or frozen yoghurt

1 quantity homemade chocolate sauce (page 215)

Chop the almonds into small chunks and toss in a frying pan over medium heat for 3–4 minutes, or until they are lightly toasted. Remove them from the heat and cool.

Slice each banana lengthways and place in a small serving bowl. Whip the evaporated milk in a bowl until frothy and creamy.

Spoon the ice-cream or frozen yoghurt over each of the bananas followed by a small amount of the chocolate sauce. Next, place a dollop of the whipped milk to the side of the sauce and finish with a sprinkle of the toasted almonds.

Serve immediately.

1 Serve: 9g total fat • 3g saturated fat • 1016kJ (242 calories) • 39g carbohydrates • 7g protein • 5g fibre

Chocolate Blackforest Sundaes

Blackforest is associated with a very rich chocolate and cherry cake laced with liquor. This sundae is based on the blackforest flavours but contains no cake or liquor and only a very small amount of chocolate. It would work just as well with cherries when they are in season.

Serves: 4 • **Makes**: 4 sundaes • **Difficulty**: easy • **Takes**: 10–15 minutes to prep

1 teaspoon cornflour
415g tin cherries in syrup
8 tablespoons low-fat chocolate ice-cream or no-fat Greek yoghurt
1 tablespoon good quality chocolate bits

Mix the cornflour with a teaspoon of the cherry syrup. Set aside.

Place the cherries and ¼ cup (60ml) of the syrup in a small saucepan. Heat gently until bubbles begin to form on the surface, then add the cornflour mixture. Stir until the mixture turns clear. Allow to cool.

Place the ice-cream in four sundae bowls. Pour over the cherry sauce.

Sprinkle the chocolate bits over the cherries and ice-cream. Serve immediately.

For a food nerd: Use the no-fat Greek yoghurt instead of the ice-cream.

1 Serve: 4g total fat • 0.5g saturated fat • 1378kJ (328 calories) • 58g carbohydrates • 17g protein • 3g fibre

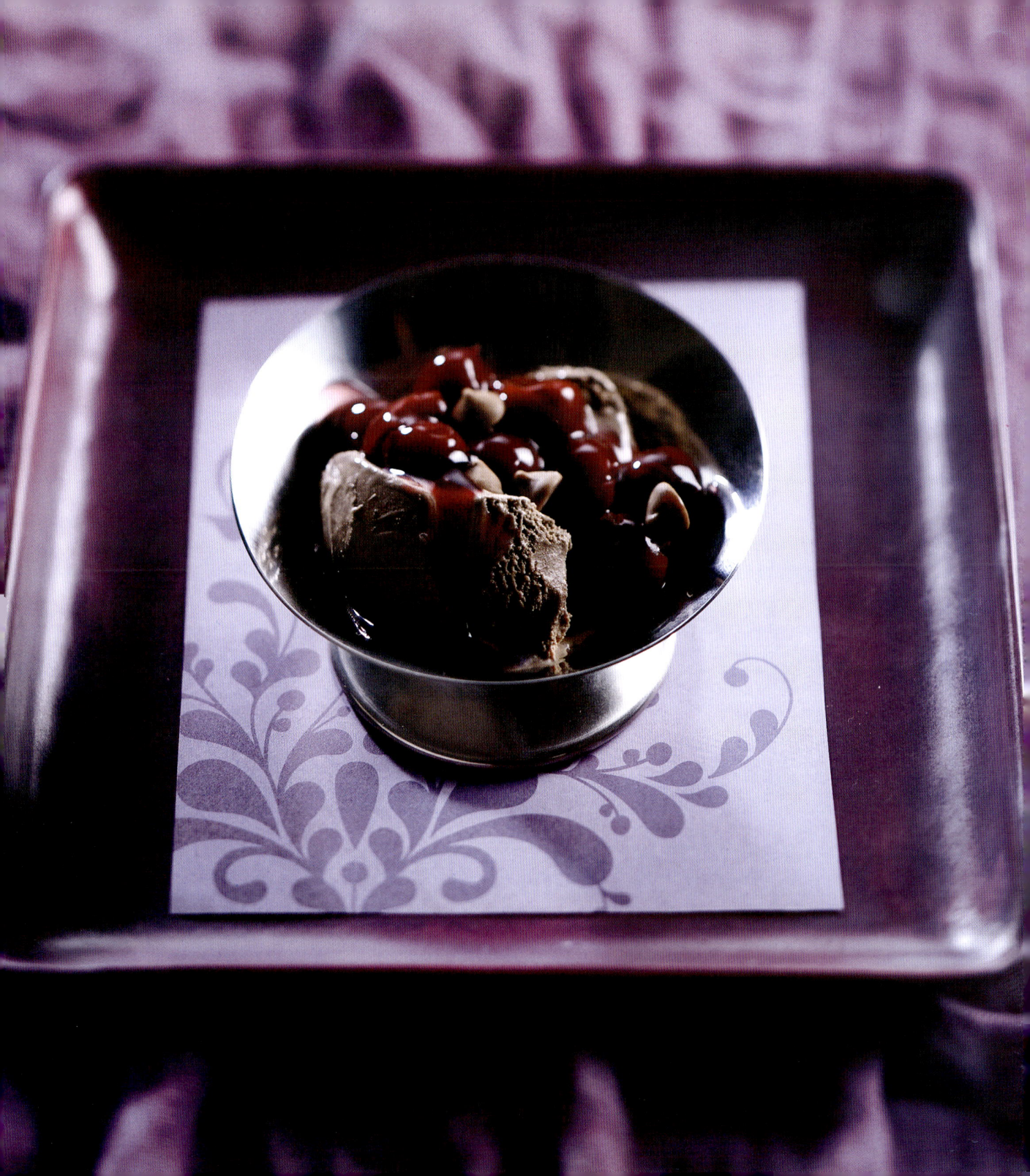

Banana Ice-cream

This is like old-fashioned ice-cream made with milk not cream. It can be made with or without an ice-cream machine. Taste it at the whipping stage to see if it is sweet enough for you, as it had been made with a minimal amount of sugar. Add a little more if required — just a little …

Serves: 6 • **Makes:** Approximately 2 cups (500ml) • **Difficulty:** easy • **Takes:** 10–15 minutes to prep, 15 minutes to cool, 3 hours to freeze

2½ cups (625ml) low-fat evaporated milk
½ cup (125ml) skim milk powder
1 tablespoon cornflour
½ teaspoon natural vanilla extract
3 tablespoons pure maple syrup
2 large very ripe bananas*
½ cup (110g) sugar

Place all the ingredients in a food processor and pulse to combine well.

Pour the mixture into a medium sized, heavy-based saucepan and heat gently, stirring constantly, until the mixture boils. Turn down to a simmer and stir until it thickens slightly. Set aside to cool.

If you have an ice-cream machine, pour the cooled mixture in and churn as per the manufacturer's instructions to the desired consistency.

If you do not have an ice-cream machine, pour the ice-cream into a freezer-safe container, cover and freeze until only the edges are solid (40 minutes to an hour). Remove from the freezer and use an electric mixer to beat the mixture until it is fluffy and light.

Return to the freezer and freeze until solid.

Allow the ice-cream to soften before serving.

* If you use lady finger bananas they will not brown. If they are too expensive, use normal bananas but add a teaspoon of lemon juice to stop them from browning.

1 Serve: 2.7g total fat • 2g saturated fat • 1201kJ (286 calories) • 53g carbohydrates • 17g protein • 2g fibre

Crème Anglaise (Custard)

Crème Anglaise, or English cream, is a light custard that can be used warm or cold. It is a better option than cream as an accompaniment to desserts.

Serves: 4-6 • **Makes:** 2 cups (500ml) • **Difficulty:** medium • **Takes:** 5 minutes to cook

2 egg yolks
1½ cups (375ml) skim
   milk
1 tablespoon sugar
1½ tablespoons plain or
   rice flour
3 drops natural vanilla
   extract

Beat the egg yolks in a large bowl until light and fluffy. Set aside.

Heat the milk in a saucepan over medium heat until it just begins to foam. Remove from heat.

Working quickly, add the sugar, flour and vanilla to the egg yolks and whisk until smooth.

Pour 2 tablespoons of the hot milk into the egg-yolk mixture and stir. Gradually whisk the rest of the milk into the eggs.

Return the egg mixture to the saucepan and, stirring constantly, over medium heat cook the custard until it thickens and lightly coats the back of a wooden spoon.

Remove from heat and serve the crème Anglaise hot or cold. If it thickens too much as it cools, add a small amount of milk to thin it.

Variation: If you want a thicker custard, add an extra ½ tablespoon of flour to the egg yolk and sugar mixture and cook the custard for longer until it thickens to desired consistency.

1 Serve: 1.2g total fat • 0.5g saturated fat • 218kJ (52 calories) • 7g carbohydrates • 3g protein • 0g fibre

Berry Compote

This compote is delicious, nutritious, easy to make, versatile and the simple ingredients are always on hand. It is a great way to entice non-fruit eaters to eat nutrition packed berries.

Serves: 4 • **Makes**: 1 cup (250ml) • **Difficulty**: easy • **Takes**: 5 minutes to cook

1 teaspoon cornflour
1 cup (125g) mixed
  frozen berries, thawed
2 teaspoons caster sugar

Mix the cornflour with 1 tablespoon of water to make a thin paste. Set aside.

Place the mixed berries in a small saucepan with the caster sugar and cook over medium heat until the berries begin to release their juice.

Add the cornflour paste and stir until the sauce becomes glossy and thick.

Serving suggestions: You can mix the compote through natural low-fat yoghurt, serve it on a cake in place of icing, as a side dish or even as a dipping sauce for fresh fruit.

1 Serve: 0g total fat • 0g saturated fat • 126kJ (30 calories) • 7.5g carbohydrates • 0.3g protein • 0.8g fibre

Chocolate Sauce

A berry compote is a delicious and far healthier choice than chocolate sauce, but this recipe is included in case you are a big chocaholic, as it is a better version of chocolate sauce to use than the fat-filled traditional version.

Serves: 4 • **Makes:** ½ cup (125ml) • **Difficulty:** easy • **Takes:** 10 minutes to cook

¼ cup (60ml) low-fat milk
1 teaspoon cornflour
1 tablespoon unsweetened cocoa powder
2 heaped tablespoons brown sugar
¼ cup (60ml) water

Mix 2 teaspoons of the milk with the cornflour to make a thin paste. Set aside.

Blend the cocoa, sugar and water to a paste in a small saucepan. Add the cornflour paste and combine well. Place over medium heat and stir until boiling, then turn down to low and simmer for 5–7 minutes, stirring occasionally, until it thickens. It will thicken further as it cools.

Use sparingly, hot or cold.

1 **Serve:** 0.1g total fat • 0g saturated fat • 168kJ (40 calories) • 9g carbohydrates • 1g protein • 0.3g fibre

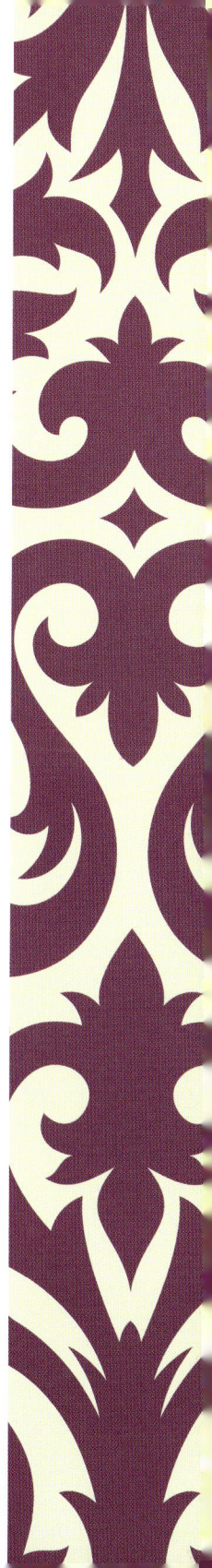

The Finishing Touches

That dollop of cream or full-fat ice-cream on the side could undo all your good work in a moment. This is not about depriving you, it is about taking a moment to think about some alternatives that will still complement your sweet treats but not add unwanted extras. Below are some tables comparing the fat of some common final touches with some of our healthier options. The recipes for crème Anglaise and custard are on page (213).

Creams per 1 tablespoon (15ml) serve:

Cream	Fat (g)
Crème fraîche	11.1
Mascarpone (cheese)	12.6
Double	15.5
Single	10.5
Light	3.6

Alternatives per 1 tablespoon (15ml) serve

Alternative	Fat (g)
Full-fat evaporated milk	1.76
Low-fat evaporated milk	0.32
Low-fat natural yoghurt	1.2
Low-fat Greek yoghurt	1.5
No-fat Greek yoghurt	.02
Low-fat ricotta cheese	1.12
Extra-light ricotta cheese	0.4
Low-fat cream cheese (80%)	3.5
Low-fat custard	0.18

Quick Cream

The evaporated milk in this dish needs to be full-fat and chilled to work well. If very cold, it will take less than a minute to double in quantity and become fluffy and creamy. It deflates quickly, so use it immediately. If you want to use it on something like a trifle where it needs to retain its volume, use the faux cream on the opposite page.

Serves 10

375ml tin full-fat evaporated milk, chilled

Whip the milk with an electric mixer until it thickens to a cream consistency.
Serve immediately.

1 Serve: 2g total fat • 1g saturated fat • 139kJ (33 calories) • 3g carbohydrates • 2g protein • 0g fibre

Faux Cream

This cream holds its volume and so can be used for sundaes, splits, trifles or any dessert that needs to sit for a while.

Serves 10

¼ cup (60ml) water

3 teaspoons powdered gelatine

375ml tin full-fat evaporated milk, chilled

2 teaspoons icing sugar

1 teaspoon natural vanilla extract

In a small saucepan, bring the water to the boil. Reduce to a simmer and sprinkle the gelatine over the water. Stir until the gelatine completely dissolves. This takes less than a minute. Remove from heat.

Whip the milk with an electric mixer until it thickens to a cream consistency. With the beaters still on, add the icing sugar and vanilla, then slowly pour in the warm gelatine mixture. Whip for a further 30 seconds, then scrape down the side of the bowl and whip for a final 30 seconds until fluffy and well combined.

Refrigerate and use cold in place of whipped cream.

1 Serve: 2g total fat • 1g saturated fat • 139kJ (33 calories) • 3g carbohydrates • 2g protein • 0g fibre

Ricotta Cream

This tastes richer than the evaporated-milk-based creams and is very nice alongside fruit pies and fruit-based desserts.

Serves 4

⅓ cup (90g) low-fat cream cheese

⅓ cup (90g) extra low-fat ricotta

½ teaspoon natural vanilla extract

2 teaspoons skim milk

2 tablespoons icing sugar

Whisk all the ingredients together and serve in a bowl cold.

1 Serve: 0.3g total fat • 0.2g saturated fat • 361kJ (86 calories) • 16g carbohydrates • 5g protein • 0g fibre

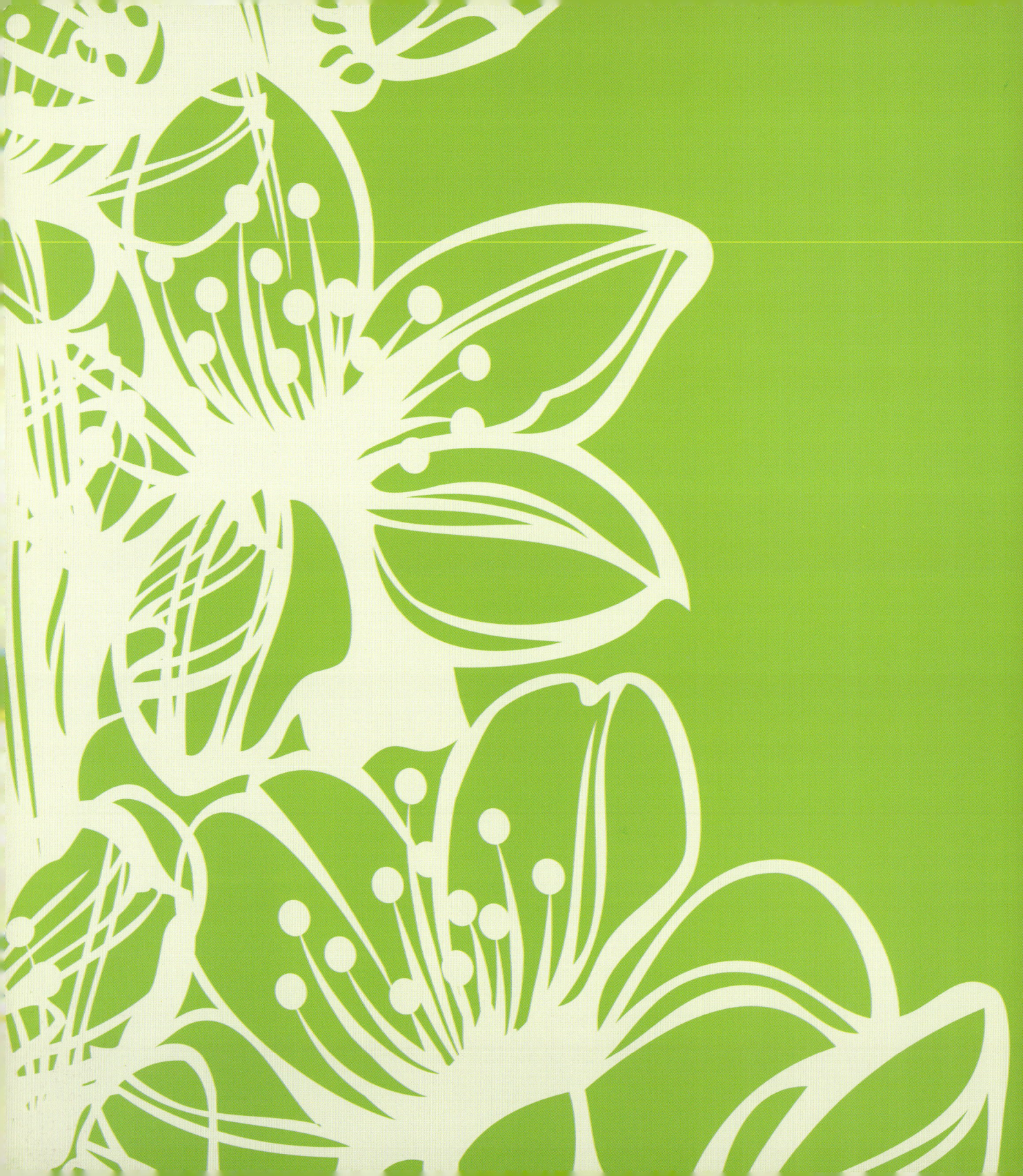

Fab Drinks

Drinks can be a lovely way to relax, whether it's with friends, your partner or your children, you can sit and have a good old chat over a drink. Samantha Stevens was a fantastic drink fixer in Bewitched. She even had a dedicated drinks' trolley. It's rather old fashioned these days as most of us just open a bottle rather than taking the time to mix or make a drink.

Fixing yourself a delicious drink gives you a sense of occasion and makes you stop and take a break from your chaotic life to sit and enjoy it rather than guzzle it down and charge on.

The drinks in this chapter are low in fat but some still hold a few calories, so if you are watching your weight, skip these few and stay with the low-calorie options, they are just as delicious.

The only alcohol in these mockatinis is the minute amount in the rum extract used in the pina colada. Aside from this, they are entirely alcohol free but taste like the real thing, they only have a fraction of the kilojoules and fat; and they look very fancy! Even Samantha would be impressed.

Iced Chocolate

It may seem like a lot of work to whip evaporated milk just for a drink but it takes only a couple of minutes and is worth it for this iced chocolate and the iced coffee that follows. When you drink it, your first taste is of the creaminess of the whipped milk and then you get the chocolate flavour.

Makes: 4 iced chocolates • **Difficulty:** easy • **Takes:** 10 minutes to prep

185ml tin low-fat evaporated milk, chilled
2½ tablespoons low-fat drinking chocolate
⅓ cup (80ml) boiling water
800ml skim milk, chilled
12 ice cubes

Using an electric mixer, whip the evaporated milk until light and fluffy (1–2 minutes).

Mix the drinking chocolate with the boiling water to make a smooth paste.

Pour an equal amount of the chocolate into four heatproof glasses. Next, add the skim milk until it fills three-quarters of the glass. Add the ice cubes. Finally, spoon 2 tablespoons of the whipped evaporated milk over the top.

1 Serve: 1.2g total fat • 1g saturated fat • 596kJ (142 calories) • 23g carbohydrates • 10g protein • 0g fibre

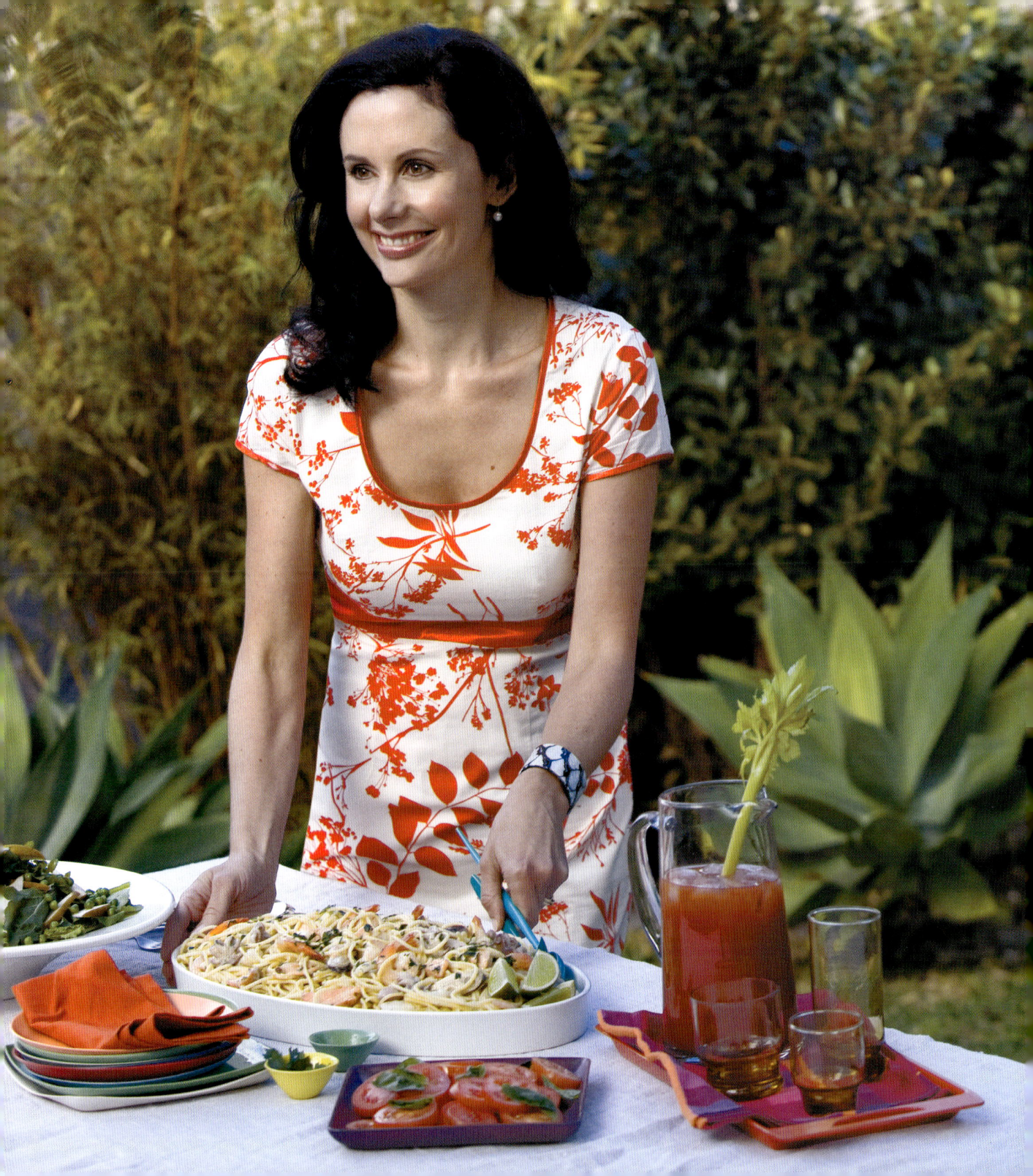

Iced Coffee

Iced coffee contains caffeine, a natural stimulant that has numerous effects on the body. For most people, it is fine in moderation but try to keep to one caffeinated drink a day.

Makes: 4 iced coffees • **Difficulty:** easy • **Takes:** 10 minutes to prep

185ml tin low-fat evaporated milk, chilled

4 teaspoons instant coffee

⅓ cup (80ml) boiling water

800ml low-fat milk, chilled

12 ice cubes

1 teaspoon sugar (if you really have to)

Using an electric mixer, whip the chilled evaporated milk until light and fluffy (1–2 minutes).

Mix the coffee and the boiling water to a smooth paste.

Pour an equal amount of the coffee into 4 glasses. Next add the low-fat milk until it fills ¾ of the glass. Add the ice cubes. Finally, spoon 2 tablespoons of the whipped evaporated milk over the top.

1 Serve: 1g total fat • 0.7g saturated fat • 441kJ (105 calories) • 16g carbohydrates • 10g protein • 0g fibre

Banana Smoothie

Throughout the book and in the meal plans I have recommended serving a smoothie. Smoothies are a great way to boost your fruit intake and add some healthy boosters like wheatgerm to your diet. Use seasonal fruit when possible. If buying a smoothie, check that the yoghurt is low-fat and that no ice-cream is added.

Serves: 2 • **Difficulty:** easy • **Takes:** 5 minutes to prep

2 cups (500ml) skim milk or unsweetened apple juice

2 bananas, roughly broken into pieces

2 tablespoons low-fat vanilla yoghurt

1 tablespoon pure maple syrup or honey

1 tablespoon wheatgerm

Place all the ingredients into a blender and blend until smooth.

Variations: For a strawberry smoothie, replace the bananas with a punnet of strawberries, washed and hulled. For a berry smoothie, replace the bananas with one cup of frozen mixed berries.

For a food nerd: If weight loss is not your goal, add 1 tablespoon of LSA (ground linseeds, sunflower seeds and almonds) and 1 egg for added protein, vitamins and minerals.

1 Serve: 1.5g total fat • 1g saturated fat • 1058kJ (252 calories) • 52g carbohydrates • 12g protein • 3.5g fibre

Pina Colada

This pina colada contains rum extract and so is not entirely alcohol free, although the amount of alcohol contained in the extract is miniscule. Some supermarkets sell alcohol-free rum extract. When buying any extract, make sure it is labelled as natural or pure. Imitation extracts and essences are cheaper and are artificial and don't have the depth or richness of flavour of the natural extracts. Extracts can be stored in a cool, dark place indefinitely.

Makes: 4 drinks • **Difficulty:** easy • **Takes:** 5 minutes to prep

1 cup (250ml) low-fat evaporated coconut-flavoured milk
1 cup (250ml) skim milk
2 cups (500ml) unsweetened pineapple juice
2 teaspoons rum extract (optional)
12 ice cubes
225g tin crushed pineapple
4 pineapple wedges, to serve

Blend all the ingredients except for the 4 pineapple wedges until the ice is completely crushed. Sieve to remove any remaining pineapple bits.
Serve with a pineapple wedge on the side of the glass.

1 Serve: 1g total fat • 0.6g saturated fat • 664kJ (158 calories) • 31.3g carbohydrates • 6.6g protein • 0.5g fibre

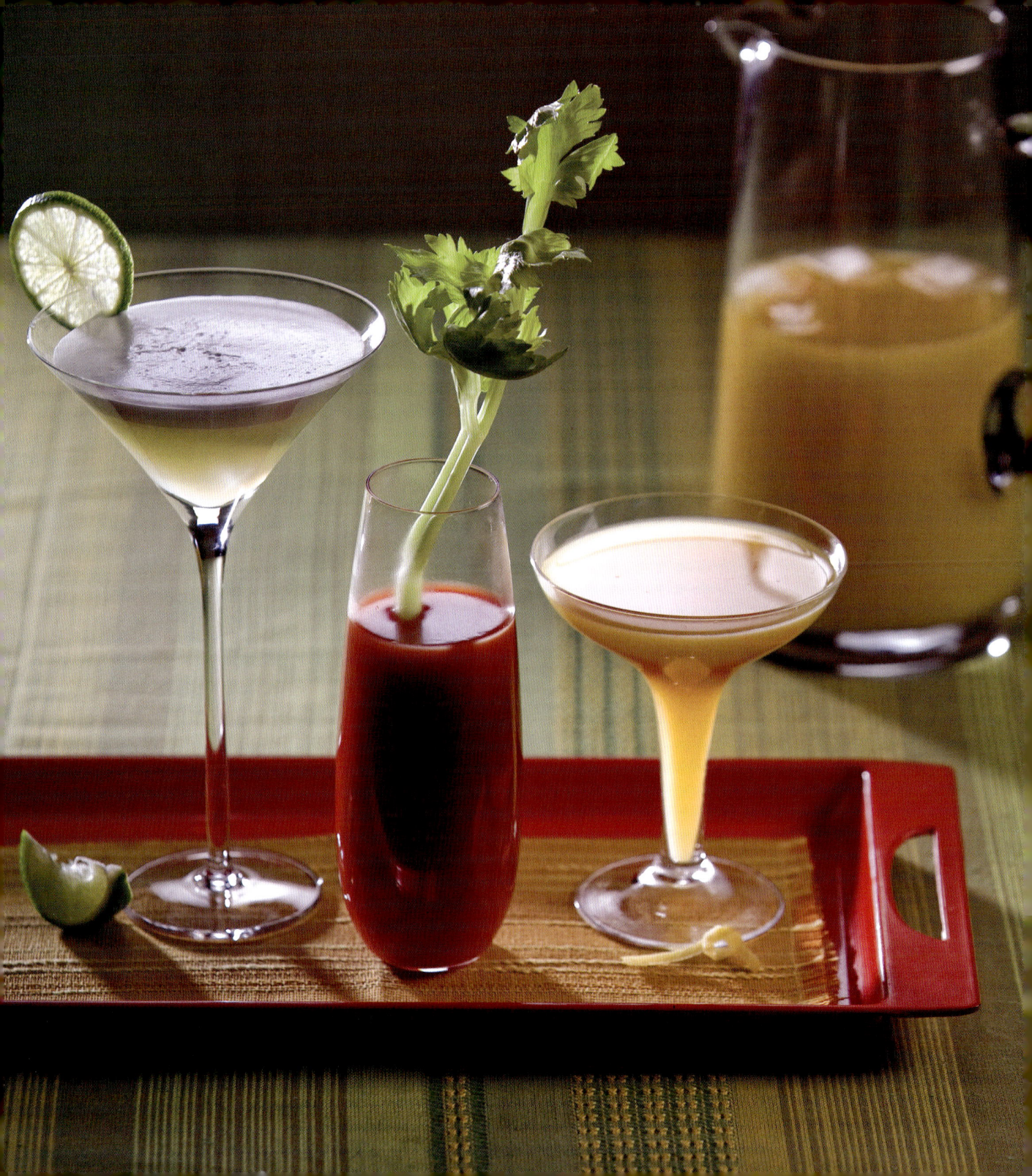

Creamy Margarita

This alcohol-free margarita is a fantastic (and surprising) inclusion in a brunch menu. It is lovely with lime sorbet and lime juice too.

Makes: 4 drinks • **Difficulty:** easy • **Takes:** 5 minutes to prep

1 cup good quality, shop-bought lemon sorbet
185ml tin low-fat evaporated milk
220ml skim milk
8 ice cubes
juice of ½ lemon
4 slices lemon, to serve

In a food processor, blend all of the ingredients except for the lemon until they are well combined.

Pour in the margarita mixture into four martini glasses and serve with a slice of lemon on the side.

1 Serve: 3.4g total fat • 2.4g saturated fat • 541kJ (129 calories) • 21.5g carbohydrates • 4.7g protein • 0g fibre

Virgin Bloody Mary

A traditional bloody Mary is already low fat and healthy but it does include vodka. This virgin variety is a great alternative to alcohol while still providing the sense of occasion that we look for when we enjoy a drink. It is also a great way to boost your vegetable intake for the day without you even knowing it.

Makes: 4 drinks • **Difficulty:** easy • **Takes:** 5 minutes to prep

2 cups (500ml) tomato juice

½ teaspoon lemon juice

2 teaspoons Worcestershire sauce

6 drops Tabasco or chilli sauce

4 lime wedges

4 celery stalks with leaves, trimmed and washed

Combine the tomato juice, lemon juice, Worcestershire sauce and Tabsaco in a jug. Stir well and pour into four long glasses.

Squeeze a wedge of lime into each drink and then drop the lime wedge into the drink.

Serve with a slim, long stalk of celery in each drink.

1 Serve: 0.1g total fat • 0g saturated fat • 88kJ (21 calories) • 5g carbohydrates • 1g protein • 0.5g fibre

A thirst for fat – an insider's guide to high-calorie drinks

Drinks can be a wonderful addition to a healthy diet by boosting hydration and fruit and vegetable intake or they can be a source of hidden disaster. Interestingly, some published Danish studies have found that sugar in drinks is more likely to produce weight gain than solid sugar in foods because the liquid sugar kilojoules don't register with the brain's satiety or fullness centre. If you are prone to gaining a few extra kilos, drinks are a good area to keep an eye on.

The right choices in drinks are not always obvious as it is surprising where sneaky kilojoules can be found. It's all about knowing what is inside your drinks so you can factor them in and make sure they are working for you – not secretly against you.

Soft drinks and juices

Looking at the table below, you can see that many soft drinks and juices are similar in the amount of energy or the amount of kilojoules they contain. But this is only one way to measure the goodness of food and drinks as the kilojoules contained in these drinks only tell half the story.

Soft drinks and pre-sweetened drinks

Drink	Kilojoules
Cola soft drink	430
Cordial (diluted)	360
Sports drink	275
Iced tea	330

Juices

Drink	Kilojoules
Apple juice	325
Orange juice	400
Carrot juice	340
Pineapple juice	440
Shop-bought fruit smoothie	675

This next table puts it into context. While the kilojoules look very similar between soft drinks and juices, the nutrients are a very different story. Soft drinks and pre-sweetened drinks offer no nutrients, only kilojoules.

Source of	Soft Drink	Carrot Juice	Orange Juice	Fruit Smoothie*
B vitamins	No	Yes	Yes	Yes
Vitamin A	No	Yes	Yes	Yes
Vitamin C	No	Yes	Yes	Yes
Magnesium	No	Yes	Yes	Yes
Potassium	No	Yes	Yes	Yes
Phosphorous	No	Yes	Yes	Yes

* This is based on an average mixed fruit smoothie bought from a popular fresh juice chain.

Alcohol

Alcohol is a potent source of kilojoules, which is clearly shown when you compare it to carbohydrate, protein and fat.

1 gram of carbohydrate = 16 kilojoules   1 gram of fat = 37 kilojoules
1 gram of protein = 16 kilojoules   1 gram of alcohol = 29 kilojoules

In terms of a standard drink, a full-strength beer has around 400 kilojoules, wine 336 kilojoules, champagne 325 kilojoules, gin and tonic 460 kilojoules, a daiquiri 750 kilojoules and the spirit premix bottles hold around 900 kilojoules! To get an idea of what this really means, you would need to walk for 30 minutes to burn off a single beer or wine, swim for 30 minutes to get rid of a daiquiri and work hard on a stair machine for 30 minutes to burn off one spirit premix bottle.

To keep on track with your healthy eating plan, you don't need to eliminate alcohol altogether, but just be aware of the amount of kilojoules or extra energy it is adding to your diet. Alcohol offers no nutrients and, in fact, uses some of our stores of vitamins and minerals to be processed. Try to have at least a couple of alcohol-free days a week and try some lower calorie alcoholic drinks, like light beer, white wine spritzers, shandies, low-calorie cocktails or non-alcoholic cocktails or mixing champagne with orange juice.

If your goal is to lose weight, eliminating alcohol until you start to reach some significant milestones will really accelerate your weight loss and so help to keep you motivated.

Lime Daiquiri

For a change you could use a mixture of lemon and orange juice to make a citrus daiquiri.

Makes: 4 drinks • **Difficulty:** easy • **Takes:** 5 minutes to prep

¼ cup (55g) sugar
¼ cup (60ml) water
¾ cup (185ml) freshly squeezed lime juice
   (about 5 limes)
4 egg whites
4 ice cubes
rind or slices of 1 lime, to serve

Make a syrup by placing the sugar and water in a small saucepan and simmering until the sugar dissolves. Allow to cool.

Blend in a food processor, the lime juice, 4 tablespoons of the sugar syrup, the egg whites and the ice until the ice is completely crushed.

Serve in a martini glass with a slice of lime on the side or a curled ribbon of lime rind in the drink.

1 Serve: 0.1g total fat • 0g saturated fat • 323kJ (77calories) • 17g carbohydrates • 5g protein • 0.2g fibre

Mock Mai Tai

This tastes like the sort of cocktail you would order on a tropical island. You could serve it in half a coconut shell and dream of sand, white beaches …

Makes: 4 drinks • **Difficulty:** easy • **Takes:** 5 minutes to prep

2 cups (500ml) fresh orange juice
1⅓ cups (330ml) pineapple juice
2 teaspoons lemon juice
2 teaspoons rum essence
4 ribbons of lemon rind

Combine all the ingredients except the lemon rind in a jug.

Serve in four martini glasses with a ribbon of lemon rind in each.

1 Serve: 0.4g total fat • 0.1g saturated fat • 424kJ (101 calories) • 24g carbohydrates • 1g protein • 0.4g fibre

Bananarama

You could use coffee essence here in place of the coffee if you like or an organic decaffeinated coffee if you don't want the caffeine. This has none of the cream of the original bananarama — or the alcohol.

Makes: 4 drinks • **Difficulty**: easy •
Takes: 5 minutes to prep

4 teaspoons instant coffee
4 teaspoons boiling water
3 frozen ripe bananas, roughly chopped
3 cups (750ml) skim milk
1 banana, skin on, thickly sliced

Blend the coffee, the boiling water, frozen banana and skim milk until smooth.

Serve in glasses garnished with a thick slice of banana on the side.

Lemon Spritzer

This is a low-sugar lemonade.

Makes: 4 drinks • **Difficulty**: easy •
Takes: 5 minutes to prep

¼ cup (55g) sugar
¼ cup (60ml) water
juice of 4 lemons
1.25 litre bottle soda water or
 mineral water

Make a syrup by placing the sugar and water in a small saucepan and simmering until the sugar dissolves. Allow to cool.

Divide the lemon juice between four glasses. Add 1½ tablespoons of the sugar syrup to each glass and top up with the soda or mineral water. Serve immediately.

1 Serve: 0.6g total fat • 0.4g saturated fat • 508kJ (121 calories) • 22g carbohydrates • 8g protein • 1.2g fibre

1 Serve: 0g total fat • 0g saturated fat • 252kJ (60 calories) • 17g carbohydrates • 0.2g protein • 0.2g fibre

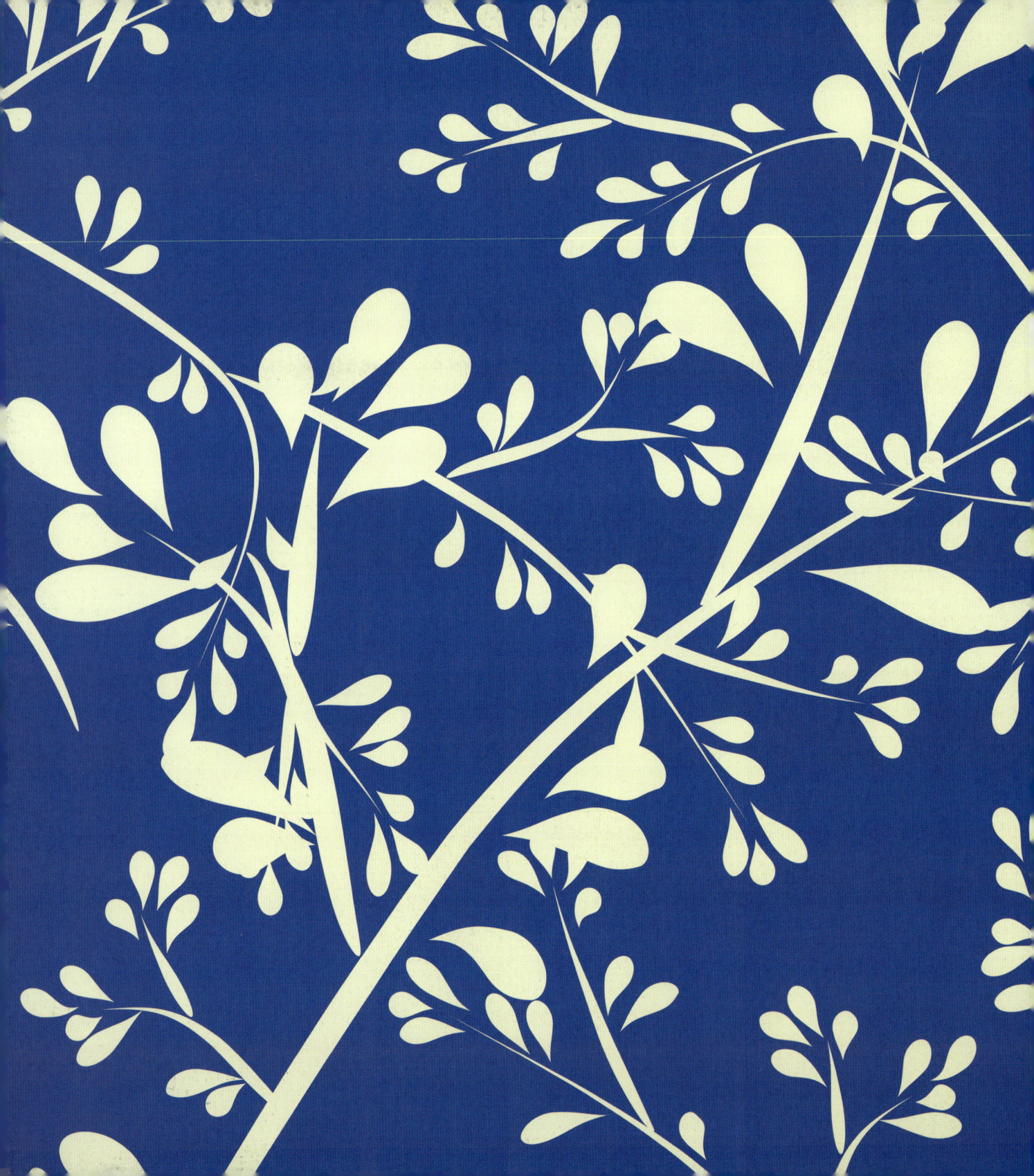

Resources

Seasonal menu plans

Quick guide to using herbs and spices

Cooking tips

A closer look at cheese

Focus on protein

Interesting books and websites

Seasonal menu plans

These menu plans are given as a guide and exact quantities are not always provided as amounts vary according to your health goals, your age, your appetite and how active you are. As menu choices and fresh food availability change depending on the time of year, there is a weekly menu plan for each season.

If you do not eat any dairy, then soy or goat products could be substituted for all dairy products in the menu plans. During autumn and winter, it is important to eat more warm foods and so the menu plans often recommend left-overs from the night before with a small alteration. Few of us have time to make a warm weekday lunch so using left-overs is an easy time-saving solution.

A week in spring

	Breakfast	Lunch	Dinner
Monday	1 cup high-fibre breakfast cereal with low-fat milk 1 sliced banana	Caesar salad	Green chicken curry with rice and cucumber raita
Tuesday	Wholegrain toast with pesto and sliced tomato Low-fat yoghurt	Hummus, salad and tuna wrap	Chicken parmigiana, potato salad and rocket
Wednesday	1 cup high-fibre breakfast cereal with low-fat milk 1 sliced banana	Left-over chicken parmigiana wholemeal sandwich with tomato, sprouts and lettuce	Garlic prawns with Chinese greens with bean sprouts and mirin Strawberry mousse
Thursday	Fresh fruit salad with low-fat ricotta, cottage cheese or low-fat yoghurt	Harissa rice salad Stewed apple with low-fat vanilla yoghurt	Bangers and mash with red salsa and beetroot, watercress and parsley salad
Friday	Corn crackers with hummus Berry fruit smoothie Wholewheat toast with avocado and sliced tomato	Chicken, lettuce, beetroot and low-fat mayonnaise sandwich Piece of fresh fruit	Grilled trout with cauliflower cheese and orange mash Vanilla panna cotta
Saturday	Apple and cinnamon pancakes	Club sandwich	Tuna mornay with rocket, pear and pea salad
Sunday	Grilled, caramelised fruits with low-fat vanilla yoghurt	Salmon salad and crackers	Nachos

A week in summer

	Breakfast	**Lunch**	**Dinner**
Monday	Fresh summer melons with low-fat ricotta cheese and pure maple syrup dipping sauce	Chicken and salad wrap Fresh fruit	Thai fish cakes with pear and parmesan salad and caprese salad
Tuesday	1 cup high-fibre breakfast cereal with low-fat milk 1 sliced banana	Left-over Thai fish cakes with rainbow salad	Lean beef steak with orange mash and green salad
Wednesday	Muesli with chopped dried apricots and apple Banana smoothie	Moroccan bean salad Tub of low-fat yoghurt	Salmon with lemon pepper crust and potato salad Apple pie with faux cream
Thursday	1 cup high-fibre breakfast cereal with low-fat milk 1 sliced banana	Sushi Dried fruit	Fried rice Fruit salad with low-fat or no-fat Greek yoghurt
Friday	Grilled pineapple with low-fat vanilla yoghurt Piece of wholegrain toast with avocado	Tuna salad sandwich Piece of fruit	Creamy scrambled eggs with Moroccan bean salad and green salad
Saturday	Eggs benedict	Tinned salmon mixed into potato salad	Wiener schnitzel with salad Banana split
Sunday	Fresh fruit salad and low-fat yoghurt	Welsh rarebit with green salad Piece of fruit	Ratatouille (from the freezer) with chickpeas and rice

A week in autumn

	Breakfast	Lunch	Dinner
Monday	1 cup high-fibre breakfast cereal with warmed low-fat milk Stewed apple	Curried egg and rocket sandwich on wholegrain bread	Vegetable pizza with garden salad
Tuesday	Stewed apple with cinnamon and low-fat or no-fat Greek yoghurt	Left-over vegetable pizza with garden salad	Lean beef steak and mixed stir-fried vegetables with mirin
Wednesday	1 cup high-fibre breakfast cereal with warmed low-fat milk Stewed apple	Cream of pumpkin soup Dried fruit and nuts	Spicy fried chicken with orange mash and tamari cauliflower and broccoli
Thursday	Baked beans on wholegrain toast	Chicken and salad wrap Low-fat yoghurt	Grilled tuna with orange mash and Chinese greens with bean sprouts and mirin Crème caramel
Friday	Stewed apple with cinnamon and low-fat or no-fat Greek yoghurt	Sushi Fruit smoothie	Green chicken curry
Saturday	Waffles with berry compote and low-fat ricotta	Vegetable soup	Pie and chips with fresh asparagus and coleslaw
Sunday	Fry up	Cream of pumpkin soup	Garden salad with warmed chicken tossed through and a fab dressing

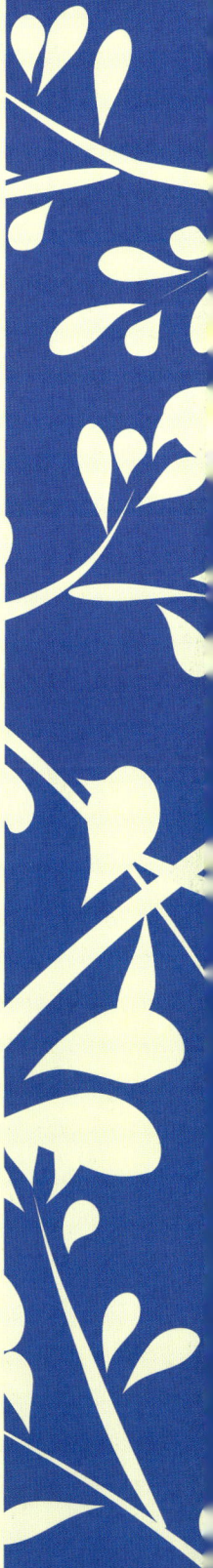

A week in winter

	Breakfast	Lunch	Dinner
Monday	Porridge	Cream of leek and potato soup	Green chicken curry
Tuesday	Creamy scrambled eggs with wholegrain toast	Rice crackers Left-over chicken green curry	Chilli con carne with Chinese greens and bean sprouts on the side
Wednesday	1 cup high-fibre breakfast cereal with low-fat milk Stewed apple	Tuna and mixed greens sandwich with lemon juice and low-fat mayonnaise Vegetable soup Wholegrain bread	Grilled salmon with orange mash and tamari cauliflower and broccoli
Thursday	Porridge	Vegetable soup Wholegrain bread	Hearty beef stew
Friday	1 cup high-fibre breakfast cereal with low-fat milk	Toasted chicken and red salsa sandwich Carrot and beetroot juice	Hawaiian and vegetable pizzas
Saturday	Spanish omelette	Cream of pumpkin soup Wholemeal roll	Sausage rolls and sauce with warm steamed vegetables and green salsa for dipping
Sunday	French toast with pure maple syrup	Grilled tomato and chicken sandwich with low-fat mozzarella	Vegetable soup (from the freezer)

As you can see, snacks have not been included in the menu plans. Healthy snack ideas do not vary greatly by season (apart from seasonal fruit and vegetables), so here is a year round list to choose from. Keep snacks small and only have them if you are truly hungry and need the extra energy or blood sugar balance.

- Small tub low-sugar low-fat yoghurt
- Small handful of raw, unsalted nuts, such as almonds, walnuts, pecans, cashews
- Piece of fresh seasonal fruit
- Frozen berries, bananas or grapes in summer
- Vegetable sticks with a dip such as hummus, tzatziki or babaghanoush
- Cracker with avocado or salsa
- Homemade dried fruit balls
- Low-salt, naturally flavoured rice crackers
- Small tin of low-salt baked beans
- Trail mix of nuts, seeds and dried fruit
- Mixed seeds, such as sunflower and pepitas
- Miso soup
- Small tin of four bean mix

Quick guide to using herbs and spices

Herb	Great with...
Basil	Pesto, salads, tomato, potato salad.
Bay leaves	Soups, stews, sauces. Remove before serving.
Chervil	Salads, to garnish soups and creamy sauces.
Chives	Salads, egg dishes and to garnish soups.
Coriander	Most Asian, Mexican and Moroccan cuisines.
Dill	Smoked salmon, salads, fish.
Fennel	Curries, salads, stir-fries, casseroles.
Lemongrass	Asian cooking and stir-fries.
Mint	Lamb, potatoes, peas, fruit salad, drinks, teas and garden salads.

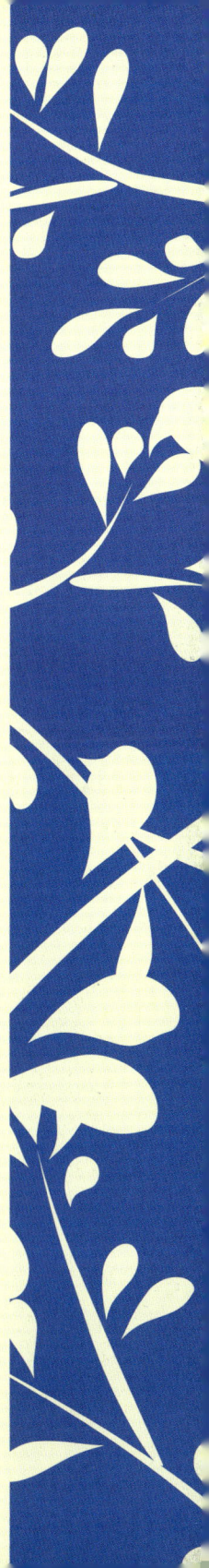

Herb	Great with...
Oregano	All Italian cooking, stuffings, egg dishes, roasts and in salads.
Parsley	In all cooking and for garnishing.
	Flat-leaf parsley is more robust and better for cooking than curly parsley. Use fresh curly parsley in salads and as a garnish.
Rosemary	Marinades, with lamb, chicken and for roasting with fish and potatoes.
Sage	Stuffings, casseroles and meat dishes.
Tarragon	Sauces, vinegars and chicken dishes.
Thyme	Italian cooking and in stews and casseroles.
Fines herbes: (Chervil, chives, parsley and French tarragon)	Fish, salads, egg dishes, chicken and sauces.
Bouquet garni: (thyme, bay leaf, parsley)	Soups, stocks, casseroles, stews. Remove from the dish before serving.
Herbes de Provence: (oregano, rosemary, marjoram, basil, bay, thyme)	Stews, pizzas, sauces and with tomatoes.

Spice	Great with...
All-spice, ground	Cakes, cookies, fruit pies, meatballs or with asparagus, chicken, tomato soups and carrots.
Caraway seeds, ground	Potato salad, cheese dishes, sauerkraut, meat marinades, lamb stew, poultry stuffing and pastry for meat pies. Sprinkle on green beans, squash, cucumbers, omelettes or tuna casserole.
Cardamom, ground	North African, Asian, and Indian cooking and in cheesecake, gingerbread, spiced cakes, with meaty sauces and chicken.
Chinese five spice	Asian stir-fries, soups, meat marinades and sauces or with meats and chicken.
Cinnamon, ground	Pies, stewed fruit and compotes, puddings, pancakes, chocolate cake, French toast, porridge or with carrots and pork.

Spice	Great with...
Cloves, ground	Apple sauce, gingerbread, stewed fruits, dessert sauces or with green vegetables.
Cumin, ground	Indian cooking, chicken, lentil, pea or bean soups, salad dressings, tomato sauces, beef stew and curry dishes.
Curry powder	Any curries, curried eggs.
Fennel seed	Salad dressing, soups, marinades or with beans, Brussel sprouts or broccoli.
Garam Masala	Indian cooking.
Ginger, ground	Cakes, cookies, gingerbread, fruit, or steamed puddings, or with chicken, beef, pork, lamb, carrots, sweet potatoes.
Nutmeg, ground	Cakes (especially pumpkin pie and carrot cake), puddings, cookies and fruit dishes.
Paprika	Red pasta sauces or with potatoes, fish or eggs.
Turmeric, ground	Curries, creamy sauces, rice, scrambled eggs, relishes and pickles or with chicken.

Cooking tips

There are some simple techniques included in the recipes that can be made even easier by using the following tips. These tips will also be useful to help ensure success when you are adapting your own recipes. Following them can make the difference between a good result and a great result for many recipes.

Egg hints

Beating egg whites

- Egg whites beat best when they are at room temperature. They will still whip straight from the fridge, but it will take longer.

- Make sure that the bowl is scrupulously clean. Stainless steel or copper bowls are best. If using a plastic bowl, give it a quick wipe out with some white vinegar or lemon juice before using it. Any traces of oil or fat will stop the whites from whipping well. Fat includes egg yolk, so always crack each egg white into a cup before adding it to the bowl. That way, if you do accidently get some egg yolk into your white, you will not have ruined all the other egg whites. This also works in case you get a rotten egg.

- If you are making a meringue and need to add sugar to the egg whites, beat the egg whites first to a soft peak before adding any sugar. A soft peak is when you take the beater or whisker out and a peak of egg white will come up with the beater but gently collapse back down once the beater is removed.

- If making meringue, add the sugar slowly. Each time you add some sugar, whip it into the egg whites well. When all the sugar is added, rub a small amount of the mixture between your finger and thumbs. If you can still feel the grittiness of the sugar, you need to keep whipping until it feels completely smooth. If you bake the pavlova or meringues with the grittiness, they will begin to weep after cooling.

- Beat the whites until they form stiff peaks. This means that if you take the beaters or the whisk out, a peak of egg white stays pointy.

Using extra yolks or whites

- If you are making a crème caramel, custard or other egg-yolk-rich delight, you will have numerous left-over egg whites. Use the whites for meringues, pavlova, in a smoothie or make egg-white poached eggs, scrambled eggs or Spanish omelette.

- Likewise, if you are making egg-white rich dishes, such as meringues, you will have left-over yolks to use. Making a baked custard is the easiest way to use them up, but be wary of how many egg yolks you use as the yolks are the source of fat and cholesterol in an egg.

Egg shell

- Always crack your eggs gently on a flat surface. This makes them crack more evenly, leaving less sharp pieces to fall into your cooking than if you crack them on the side of the bowl.

- If you do get some shell in your bowl, using the intact shell is the easiest way to retrieve it.

Blind baking

- Blind baking means partly baking a pie or pastry crust without the filling. It helps to ensure you end up with a nice crispy crust.

- To retain the shape of the case during the baking, cover the case with baking paper and weigh it down with pie weights, uncooked rice or uncooked legumes.

- Bake at 190°C–200°C for 10 minutes. Remove the weights and baking paper and reduce the temperature to 180°C. Continue baking for a further 15–20 minutes. The goal of blind baking is to seal the pastry and so protect it from becoming soggy once the filling is poured in. It will be completely cooked once it has been filled and placed back in the oven.

- If you are not using the pastry immediately, store it in an airtight container.

Baking in a water bath

- Custard and some other fragile desserts need to be baked gently and so are cooked in a water bath (bain marie).

- Place the pudding basin or ovenproof dish into the water bath dish, an empty lasagne dish or baking pan works very well. Pour boiling water into the water bath dish to fill it to two-thirds of its capacity and place immediately in the oven.

- Using water that has just boiled ensures that the pudding or custard begins to cook as soon as it is placed in the oven.

Measuring brown sugar

- To measure brown sugar accurately, it needs to be packed well down. This means you need to press it into the measuring cup so it is firmly packed. If you don't do this, it could considerably affect the outcome of your recipe, particularly if you are baking.

Pancake perfection

- Let the batter stand for around 20 minutes to activate the gluten. Don't have the pan too hot, otherwise the pancake may not cook right through before it browns. Don't use too much mix for each pancake; keep them thin so they cook right through.

- Don't overmix the batter or you will get rubbery pancakes, and don't impatiently push down on the pancake with the eggflip (why do we love to do that?) as you will push out all of the fluffiness.

Adjusting recipes to meet your individual needs

- When cooking for just one, you may not want to cook the entire recipe and when cooking for six you may need to add extra to feed the entire family. Most recipes are filled with fractions and so can be tricky to adjust correctly. Use the table below to convert the recipes to meet your individual needs.

- To use the table, look at the number of people the original recipe serves. If the original recipe serves four but you want to make it for one person, use the quarter column to convert.

- If the original recipe serves four and you want to make it for two people, use the half column to halve every measure in the recipe.

- If the original recipe serves four and you are cooking for six, then use the one and a half column.

- If the original recipe serves four and you are cooking for eight, then use the double column.

Measure*	Quarter size of recipe	Half size of recipe	One and a half times the recipe	Double the recipe
½ teaspoon	⅛ teaspoon	¼ teaspoon	¾ teaspoon	1 teaspoon
1 teaspoon	¼ teaspoon	½ teaspoon	1½ teaspoons	2 teaspoons
2 teaspoons	½ teaspoon	1 teaspoon	3 teaspoons	4 teaspoons
½ tablespoon	½ teaspoon**	1 teaspoon**	¾ tablespoon	1 tablespoons
1 tablespoon	¼ tablespoon	½ tablespoon	1½ tablespoons	2 tablespoons
2 tablespoons	½ tablespoon	1 tablespoon	3 tablespoons	4 tablespoons
¼ cup	1 tablespoon	2 tablespoons	⅜ cup or 6 tablespoons	½ cup
⅓ cup	1½ tablespoon	2½ tablespoons	½ cup	⅔ cup
½ cup	⅛ cup	¼ cup	¾ cup	1 cup
¾ cup	3 tablespoons	6 tablespoons	1⅛ cups	1½ cups
1 cup	¼ cup	½ cup	1½ cups	2 cups
2 cups	½ cup	1 cup	3 cups	4 cups
100 grams	25 grams	50 grams	150 grams	200 grams
200 grams	50 grams	100 grams	300 grams	400 grams
400 grams	100 grams	200 grams	600 grams	800 grams
500 grams	125 grams	250 grams	750 grams	1000 grams or 1 kilogram

*1 tablespoon equals 15ml which is equivalent to 3 teaspoons.

**This is not a mistake! One tablespoon is equal to 3 teaspoons so when dividing tablespoons it is easier to work it out in teaspoons.

A closer look at cheese

There is a huge difference between the fat and the fab cheeses that appear in this book. There is also great variation between brands, so always check the labels carefully before you buy.

Have a look at the table below to see where your favourite sits and get to know all the fab cheeses that are kind to your tastebuds, your heart and your hips.

The fat

Unfortunately the hard, yellow cheeses and the very soft, aged cheese with a crust never make the cut.

	Serving*	Kilojoules	Fat	Sodium
Cheddar	30g	500	10g	176mg
Brie	30g	400	8g	178.5mg
Camembert	30g	357	7g	238.5mg
Blue	30g	420	8g	395.5mg
Edam	30g	424	8g	273.5mg

*30g = 1 thick slice of cheese

The fab

A fab cheese is low in fat, calories and has relatively low salt. The softer, unaged cheeses are usually the fab ones as they have a higher water content, although they are lower in protein, nutrients and calcium. To offset this, we usually eat more of these when using them in cooking and salads.

	Serving*	Kilojoules	Fat	Sodium
Low-fat ricotta	40g	311	5g	40mg
Low-fat mozzarella	40g	302	4.5g	132mg
Low-fat cottage (1%)	40g	189	2g	114mg
Quark (2%)	40g	122	0.1g	0mg
Low-fat cream cheese (80% reduced)	40g	292	5.6g	104mg
Bocconcini	40g	342	6.1g	112mg

*40g = approximately ½ to 1 tablespoon depending on the type of cheese.

Focus on protein

The table below is included to give you an indication of the amount of protein in protein-rich foods.

Food	Grams of protein
Almonds, 28g	4.6
Baked beans, 220g	20
Tinned tuna, 100g	25
Chicken breast, lean beef, lean lamb, 120g	20
Chickpeas, ½ cup	7.25
Cow's milk, 1 cup	8
Cow's milk skim, 1 cup	8.4
Fish, 160g fillet	20
Egg, whole	6.1
Egg white	3.4
Hard cheese, 30g	7
Kidney beans, 1 cup	13.3
Pepitas, 28g	7.0
Potato, 1 baked	4.7
Ricotta cheese low-fat, 60g	7
Soy beans, ½ cup	14.3
Soy milk, 1 cup	5–10
Sunflower seeds, 28g	6.5
Tofu, 90g	7–10
Yoghurt, natural, ½ cup	3.9
Yoghurt, natural, skim, ½ cup	10

Plant protein

Plant protein is the main source of protein for many cultures, yet in the Western world it has a hippy label with few people taking advantage of its wonderful benefits. Many people don't know how to use it in their food and so here is some information on legumes and pulses and lots of ideas for boosting them in your new fab diet.

What are legumes and pulses?

Pulses are the seeds of leguminous plants. Some pulses we eat dried (cannellini beans, navy beans, lentils, split peas, etc.) and some we eat fresh (peas, snake beans and green beans).

Why are legumes and pulses so good for you?

Most of them are an excellent source of protein and are rich in vitamins and minerals. Soy beans, for example, are rich in vitamin E, folate, selenium and potassium and chickpeas are rich in iron and calcium.

Where do you get pulses?

Pulses are available from supermarkets and health food shops, either tinned or dried in packets.

How do you prepare pulses?

Preparation time depends on the pulse. A table outlining the soaking and cooking times of the more common pulses is below. If you are short on time, use the tinned versions with no added salt or sugar and always wash and drain thoroughly, before you use them in your cooking. Many supermarkets now carry organic tinned pulses and legumes, which are very reasonably priced. These are an excellent option.

Although some of the soaking and cooking times seem long, all you have to do is leave them to soak in water, drain and boil them, and so they take little of your actual time. Pulses and legumes have an infamous reputation for giving you gas, but you can help to reduce gas formation by changing the soaking and cooking water a couple of times or adding some lemon juice to the cooking water. When you change the water, you will notice it is quite smelly – this is the undesirable gases being released into the water. One more tip to remember is that whenever you cook pulses never add salt as this stops the pulses from softening.

Soak and cook a whole packet at a time and freeze it in smaller quantities to use when needed.

For cooking, all pulses and legumes need twice their own volume of water, so if you are cooking 1 cup of soy beans, you will need to cook them in 2 cups of water. Remember to start cooking with a fast boil for 10 minutes, then reduce it to a slow boil for all pulses and legumes, except split peas and lentils. It may all sound a little daunting but it is easy once you have done it a couple of times.

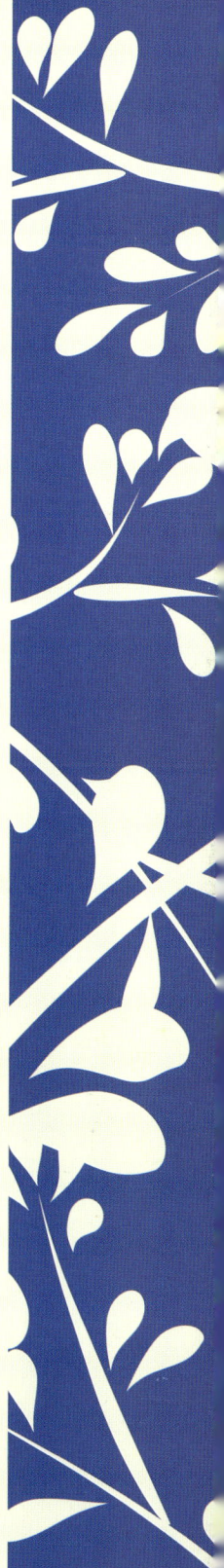

Preparation of legumes and pulses

Legume/Pulse	Soaking time	Cooking time
Soy beans	Soak overnight	2–2½ hours
Chickpeas	Soak overnight	1½ hours
Kidney beans	Soak overnight	50 minutes
Butter beans	Soak overnight	1½ hours
Haricot beans	Soak overnight	1 hour
Adzuki beans	Soak overnight	40 minutes
Split peas	No soaking	40 minutes
Red lentils	No soaking	20 minutes
Brown lentils	No soaking	20 minutes
Green lentils	No soaking	20 minutes

How do you use legumes and pulses?

Legume/Pulse	Easy ideas on how to use them
Brown lentils	In pasta sauces, stews, casseroles, soups and burgers.
Red lentils	In soups, stocks, stews, casseroles, pasta sauces. Cooked in with rice.
Chickpeas	In hummus, stews, soups, pasta sauces, casseroles, salads, curries, mashed potato. Also comes as a flour (called gram flour or besan flour and is used a lot in Indian cooking). The flour can be used in fritters and batters.
Butter beans and haricot beans	In mashed potato, soups, stews, casseroles, burgers, salads, pasta sauces, fritters and pancake batter.
Adzuki beans and kidney beans	In stews, pasta sauces, casseroles, salads.

Interesting books and websites

Books

Simply Healthy by Sally James (J.B. Fairfax Press, Sydney, 1999)
Fresh & Healthy by Sally James (J.B. Fairfax Press, Sydney, 2000)
Both of these books are the Victor Chang Research Institute cookbooks. They are filled with healthy recipes that actually look delicious, not dry and boring like so many health cookbooks.

You Are What You Eat Cookbook by Gillian McKeith (Penguin Books, London, 2005)
This is the cookbook from Gillian's brash TV show of the same name. I love it but remember that I am a self-confessed food nerd. This book is not for the faint hearted. Full of recipes filled with quinoa, seaweed and millet, it is extreme but delicious nutrition. If you are looking to push the boundaries, this one is for you.

Garden Feast by Melissa King (ABC Books, Sydney, 2007)
This inspiring book, written by a passionate gardener and foodie, shows how to grow, harvest and cook up your harvest into delicious delights. Lots of great information on unusual and heirloom varieties of fruits and vegetables.

Websites

The Complete Food Makeover
www.thecompletefoodmakeover.com.au
The book's website is filled with extra recipes, tips, ideas, videos and blogs.

Go for 2&5
www.gofor2and5.com.au/
The 2&5 website is loaded with ideas, recipes, programs and news about healthy eating. You can also sign up for their regular email newsletter. Very user-friendly.

Measure Up
www.measureup.gov.au/internet/abhi/publishing.nsf
Measure Up is an Australian Government initiative to help Australians lose weight. If weight loss is your goal, this is a great site as it is filled with excellent resources including diet diaries and eating guidelines.

Nutrition Australia
www.nutritionaustralia.org/
This site is filled with ideas and in-depth nutrition information. It also has lots of practical ideas and fact sheets on increasing variety and other easy ways to give your diet a boost.

Ministry of Health Nutrient Reference Values

www.nrv.gov.au/

This website offers in-depth nutritional information for those wanting to dig a little deeper.

Get Moving

www.healthyactive.gov.au/getmoving

Another Australian Government website dedicated to giving you lots of ideas and inspiration for healthy living.

Healthy Weight website

www.healthyactive.gov.au/internet/healthyactive/Publishing.nsf/Content/healthyweight

This website is filled with ideas about healthy eating, active lifestyles and all you need to maintain a healthy weight.

Kitchen Garden Foundation

www.kitchengardenfoundation.org.au/

The Kitchen Garden Foundation is a wonderful initiative from Stephanie Alexander. It works to set up kitchens and kitchen gardens in schools to promote a healthy diet for our children from seed to plate. A fantastic website if you are feeling inspired and want to spread the word about great food to our little guys.

Eat Well Plate

www.eatwell.gov.uk/healthydiet/eatwellplate/

The Eat Well Plate is a section on the UK's Food Standards Agency's wonderful website. It is a plate showing, in pictures, how to balance the different sorts of food you eat. It has an excellent printable version and is well worth a look. You could also take the 21-day sat fat challenge or have a look at their food mythbusting section.

How are the kids?

www.howarethekids.com/

This is another UK Government site. It is part of their Change 4 Life program. Although some of it is UK based, it is a wonderful user-friendly and engaging resource that will give you lots of tools and ideas to check your kids' diet, health and wellbeing, and how to improve them. Excellent website.

Index

The ABC 'Wave' device is a trademark of the Australian Broadcasting Corporation and is used under licence by HarperCollins*Publishers* Australia.

First published in Australia in 2011
by HarperCollins*Publishers* Australia Pty Limited
ABN 36 009 913 517
harpercollins.com.au

HarperCollins*Publishers*
25 Ryde Road, Pymble, Sydney, NSW 2073, Australia
31 View Road, Glenfield, Auckland 0627, New Zealand
A 53, Sector 57, Noida, UP, India
77–85 Fulham Palace Road, London W6 8JB, United Kingdom
2 Bloor Street East, 20th floor, Toronto, Ontario M4W 1A8, Canada
10 East 53rd Street, New York NY 10022, USA

National Library of Australia Cataloguing-in-Publication data:

Wood, Julie Maree.
    The complete food makeover / Julie Maree Wood.
    ISBN: 978 0 7333 2864 0 (pbk.)
    Includes index.
    Low-fat diet – Recipes. Cooking.
641.56384

Cover photographs by Joe Filshie
All internal photographs by Joe Filshie (www.joefilshie.com.au),
    except for pages 16, 24, 35, 117, 137, 139, 145, 164 supplied by Shutterstock.com;
    and pages 31, 36, 53 supplied by istockphoto.com. Decorative borders supplied
    by Shutterstock.com
Photographic styling: Georgie Dolling
Home economist: Jo Forrest
Book and cover design: Christa Moffitt, Christabella Designs
Typeset by Kirby Jones
Colour reproduction by Graphic Print Group
Printed by RR Donnelley in China on 128gsm Matt Art

5 4 3 2   18 19 20